Regaining
Bladder Control

Regaining
Bladder Control

What Every Woman Needs to Know

Rebecca G. Rogers, MD

Janet Yagoda Shagam, PhD

Shelley Kleinschmidt

Foreword by Ingrid Nygaard, MD

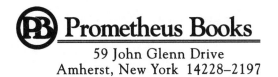

Prometheus Books

59 John Glenn Drive
Amherst, New York 14228–2197

Published 2006 by Prometheus Books

Inquiries should be addressed to
Prometheus Books
59 John Glenn Drive
Amherst, New York 14228–2197
VOICE: 716–691–0133, ext. 207
FAX: 716–564–2711
WWW.PROMETHEUSBOOKS.COM

10 09 08 07 06   5 4 3 2 1

Library of Congress Cataloging-in-Publication Data

Rogers, Rebecca G. (Rebecca Glenn), 1959–
    Regaining bladder control : what every woman needs to know / by Rebecca G.
Rogers, Janet Yagoda Shagam, and Shelley Kleinschmidt.
        p. cm.
    Includes bibliographical references and index.
    ISBN 13: 978–1–59102–416–3 (pbk. : alk. paper)
    ISBN 10: 1–59102–416–1 (pbk. : alk. paper)
    1. Urinary incontinence—Popular works. 2. Women—Diseases—Popular works.
I. Shagam, Janet Yagoda. II. Kleinschmidt, Shelley. III. Title.

RC921.I5R64 2006
616.6'2—dc22

                                                                    2006008264

Printed in the United States of America on acid-free paper

CONTENTS

CHAPTER 3. GETTING ORIENTED: THE DETAILS OF URINARY INCONTINENCE 49

CHAPTER 5. GETTING THE HELP YOU WANT   **113**

CHAPTER 6. YOUR DIAGNOSIS: A PROCESS, NOT A QUICK ANSWER   137

CHAPTER 7.   RELATED PROBLEMS: PELVIC ORGAN PROLAPSE AND ANAL INCONTINENCE   169

CHAPTER 8.   TAKE CONTROL: WITH A LITTLE OUTSIDE HELP   197

CHAPTER 9. WHEN SURGERY IS YOUR BEST OPTION   **233**

CHAPTER 10. TALKING AMONG FRIENDS 275

ACKNOWLEDGMENTS

The three of us would like to thank the following individuals for their support, enthusiasm, and invaluable comments:

The University of New Mexico Health Science Center, Albuquerque, New Mexico: Ellen Craig, RN, CNM, Peggy Gurule, RN, Kathryn Brown, PT, MS, Denise Gomez, RN, Rebecca Hall, PhD, Marty Rode, CNM, Gwendy Beer, RN, Yuko Kumesu, MD, Cindi Lewis, MD, Eve Espey, MD, Sally Bachofer, MD, MS, William Rayburn, MD, Judy Kay—Administrative Assistant "extraordinaire," and University of New Mexico professional writing intern Michelle Benson.

Lovelace-Sandia Medical Center, Albuquerque, New Mexico: Dorothy Kammerer-Doak, MD.

We are also most grateful to the dozens of Women's Health Center Urogynecology patients who generously and graciously allowed us to observe and photograph their examinations, diagnostic tests, and medical treatments, and in some cases, their surgical procedures. And if that weren't enough, these women told us their stories, too.

We would like to thank the following Albuquerque, New

Mexico, community readers: Cynthia Apostalon, Margaret Chu, Sheila Doucette, Lisa Gallegos Geier, Pat Heydt, Beryl Markowitz, Suzanne Marks, Lyle Ramsey, and Nancy Wiedower.

This book developed a whole new perspective when we had the good fortune to meet a woman who belongs to a neighborhood group called "4-Hills Neighbors." Because of her enthusiasm and ability to recruit the interest of other members and their friends and relatives, we had the opportunity to learn from yet another group of women. "Thank you 4-Hills ladies!"

The authors are especially grateful to Prometheus Books for embracing this project. We appreciate Steven L. Mitchell and the Prometheus staff for providing much-valued editorial and technical expertise and for including us in many behind-the-scenes aspects of getting this book into readers' hands.

We also wish to thank our illustrators, Darby Photos and Cris Olds. Even with our propensity for giving "do it like this—do it like that" instructions, they did a magnificent job in bringing clarity to this difficult topic.

*   *   *

To my patients for their bravery and dignity; you have inspired this book. To Mary Smith who helped me and many others grow up in the operating room, I miss you. To the wonderful group of women that I have the privilege of working with, I could not have done it without all of you. To my coauthors who made clear communication possible. Most especially to my family: my parents, who still come to see my "activities"; my creative sister, Rachel; my husband, John, who believes in me no matter what; my son, Zachariah, who keeps us all smiling; and my daughter, Hannah, whose hugs and kisses have kept me going.

Rebecca Rogers, MD

First of all, I want to thank my two coauthors for their dedication and willingness to make seemingly impossible juggles with their already too full day. I must also give a tremendous round of thanks to my husband Richard and our children Joshua, Michael, Leah, and new son-in-law, Stephane, for their encouragement and patience with an often too busy wife and mother. I also wish to acknowledge Kate Vogel, who many years ago unknowingly ignited a writing spark, and Jonathan Price for his quiet advice.

Janet Yagoda Shagam, PhD

To my coauthors, it is an honor and an inspiration to work with each of you! Thank you for your expertise, humor, and collaborative spirit throughout this rewarding task. To my endlessly supportive husband, Bill, my cherished daughters Evann and Heather, my parents, family, and friends, I am deeply grateful for your encouraging words, practical help, and generosity in sharing me with this book. And, to my trusted Mentor—you know who you are—I thank you for answering the countless "sticky-note questions" that led me to this path.

Shelley Kleinschmidt, BUS

FOREWORD

A woman without bladder control issues may think that a whole book devoted to this topic is a bit much. To you I say: respect, nurture, and be in awe of your bladder. If it has worked well for you since you trained it when you were three, be appropriately grateful. This unsung organ helps you keep your place in a society that values control, and especially bladder control. As a urogynecologist, I see countless women of all ages, sizes, and backgrounds with one common denominator: the devastating experience of losing urine in public. Just last week in my clinic, I met an executive woman in her mid-forties. Since her first child was born twenty years earlier, she leaks when she coughs, sneezes, exercises, or dances. This put a damper on her enthusiasm for some pursuits, but never precipitated a mention to her doctor. Then, in the last year, on three separate occasions, while giving a presentation in a room filled with people, she experienced a sudden urge to urinate and without further warning, lost control of her whole bladder. Now, her life is altered. She feels insecure in her job, is reluctant to appear in public, wears heavy pads and dark clothes "just in case," and is afraid to seek intimacy in her relationship. An obviously smart woman, she had no idea about the workings of her bladder or what she could do to help herself. This book is for her and for all of you who want to take back your bladders.

One in three American women leak urine. Yet, while many personal health issues are now prominent in the news and media, incontinence maintains its shroud of silence. The theories about why this is so don't interest me—what interests me is lifting this veil so that women have the information they need in a format they can use. This book fits the bill.

Rebecca Rogers, MD, is one of the top educators in urogynecology today. Thanks to her writings, medical students know what incontinence is; thanks to her videos and lectures, resident physicians repair childbirth injuries better; thanks to her research, practicing physicians learn valuable pearls: Give women antibiotics after surgery for incontinence until their catheter is removed—they will suffer less. Stop doing certain types of surgery for incontinence—they don't help enough. Ask women about their sexual function in a standardized and comprehensive way—we will learn more about this valuable part of life.

Dr. Rogers teaches the teachers. In courses around the country, she instructs practicing physicians on the unique skills needed to teach the next generation of surgeons how to repair the pelvic ravages of age, childbirth, and just plain living. In this book, Dr. Rogers closes the circle and turns her considerable skill to teaching you about one of our most important organs, the bladder, and what to do when it loses control.

This book is written from a woman's perspective. Vignettes from patients and caregivers are included throughout. The topic is focused and practical. Every aspect of bladder control is touched on, from how certain foods affect it to what to expect should you find yourself in an operating room. Women reading this book will learn more about bladder control than most medical and nursing students, but they will never feel that they need an advanced degree to understand its contents.

The authors' skills complement each other perfectly: a busy, caring clinician specialized in the treatment of bladder problems, in collaboration with a top-notch educator, a down-to-earth medical writer, and a skilled illustrator. The result is a book that never preaches, always teaches, and never makes the reader feel small. The language is easy to understand but never talks down. All major concepts are described in "nondoctor" terms. Through vocabulary lists, illustrations, and explanations, readers can also choose to learn the "doctor" terms to enhance their communication with medical professionals. Along this vein, the unique worksheets in this book will solve many communication woes. I am struck by how helpful it would be for me if my patients came prepared with these thoughtful descriptions of their symptoms, expectations, and questions.

Sections on frequently asked questions really are the questions my patients ask, once they trust me enough to open up. The concerns and coping strategies shared come directly from the mouths of my patients. Yet this book is so much more than a support group. The information shared is of high quality and scientifically based. Readers need not worry whether the imparted information is true or real. The authors clearly disclose when controversy exists, and refer women to their own physicians for matters where opinion replaces fact.

This is the book I want in my office to aid my teaching efforts. This is the book I want to send to friends and family when they ask me at the tail end of a gathering, as we're putting our coats on, what to do about (whispered voice) their bladders. This is the book I highly recommend to any of you trying to regain control of your bladders.

Ingrid Nygaard, MD, MS
Professor, Department of Obstetrics and Gynecology
Assistant Dean, Clinical Research
University of Utah

CHAPTER 1

A NEW JOURNEY

*"After reading this I felt free—I felt as though
I had just been released from jail."*
An incontinent patient

A GUIDE TO REGAINING BLADDER CONTROL

This is a proud moment—you are now taking an important first step in your bladder control journey. This is not a journey you will take alone. Throughout this book, you will meet many women who understand both what it is like to have urinary incontinence and what it takes to regain continence. Through them, you will learn about the many simple things you can do at home that often make urinary incontinence manageable. You will also accompany these women as they seek medical care and undergo treatment.

Urinary incontinence is so common that, whether you realize it or not, you know many other women who are also coping with an uncooperative bladder. While this statement may surprise you, research shows that one in three women leak urine sometime during their life. Sadly enough, most women who live with bladder control difficulties never receive care for this highly treatable condition.

It is easy to understand the reasons for this. Many women believe that bladder control problems are a natural part of the aging process and not a "real" medical concern. Many others avoid the topic because they are under the impression that pills and surgery are their only treatment options. Still others, because of the stigma associated with having urinary incontinence, feel they must keep their condition a secret.

Treating urinary incontinence is important! As you may already know, living with urinary incontinence can limit your ability to socialize with friends and family. Worrying about leaks and accidents can make going to work "too much trouble." Constantly having to think about dampness and odors can make you feel unhealthy.

Lack of complete bladder control prevents many women from seeking medical care even when not feeling well. Avoiding the doctor when you are ill is not good—especially when something like an infection goes untreated or *high blood pressure* goes undiagnosed. Although, by itself, urinary incontinence is not a life-threatening condition, it does change every aspect of your life.

Ours is not a medical text. It is a tool that will help guide you in your journey to continence. Each chapter begins with a story to offer you insight and to help orient you to the chapter topic. In these stories, based on what real women have told us, you will read about the turning point—maybe one similar to your own—that prompted some of them to get treatment. Others will tell you about their first doctor appointment, their first experiences with biofeedback therapy, or their first "dry" sneeze in over a decade.

Each chapter explores a different aspect of managing and treating urinary incontinence. First, you will become familiar with the descriptive language and the "hows and whys" of urinary incontinence. Then, we invite you to try an assortment of proven self-help strategies you can do at home. If these approaches do not provide enough relief and you decide to seek medical treatment, you will read how to find local community resources and how to communicate with the range of medical professionals you may meet on the way to better bladder control.

Because the diagnostic process can sometimes feel like a "fourteen cities in fifteen days" whirlwind tour, we prepare you for this part of your journey by describing and explaining the tests and procedures your doctor may recommend for you. Treatment of your incontinence can include appointments with other medical professionals such as *physical therapists* and nurse specialists. Learning what services they offer and what role they play in your care will help you make informed decisions. If surgery proves your best route for regaining continence, you can learn about the range of procedures available and which ones are most likely to improve your particular situation.

We have also provided an assortment of useful tools such as a glossary of terms, chapter worksheets, and frequently asked questions sections. The glossary is a source of backup information that will make understanding and using new terms easier for you.

The worksheets serve several purposes. Some will help you self-assess your personal treatment goals before you arrive at the doctor's office. Others will help you to ask questions and understand your doctor's responses to them. Still other worksheets, such as the bladder diary in chapter 4, will provide important diagnostic information you and your doctor can use. Taking the time to self-reflect and evaluate your condition will help you define personal treatment goals and take note of your progress.

Doctors like it when patients ask questions. Asking questions tells them you are thinking and actively participating in your treatment. Many doctors admit that patient's questions help them improve their explanations and provide better care. The frequently asked questions found at the end of each chapter are representative of the questions patients typically ask. You can certainly ask your doctor some of these same questions—comparing your doctor's responses to those we provide will be like getting a second opinion!

YOUR AUTHORS' JOURNEY

This book, an idea that blossomed and grew over several years, is a collaboration among three friends wishing to combine their varying professional and personal perspectives. It also reflects the point of view of the many different healthcare professionals— physical therapists, nurse midwives, nurse continence specialists, and imaging specialists—you may see during your diagnosis and treatment process. Having their input helped us provide a well-rounded tour for you.

Writing this book has been an interesting journey for us as well. Learning to craft bridges between academic research and narrative reporting took us on some unexpected side trips. The nonclinicians became adept at interviewing patients and comfortable in the examination room and surgical suite as observers. The *urogynecologist* increased her repertoire of incontinence coping strategies that she now uses to help her clinic patients. The three of us also learned to appreciate the awkwardness of asking for help in locating urinary incontinence books at the local bookstore.

A delightful surprise was discovering that under the right conditions women are comfortable talking about their bladder control problems. A network of local neighborhood women generously agreed to share their stories of leaks and embarrassing moments, coping tricks, and treatment experiences with us. Many also volunteered to read what we had written to make sure that it made sense and "rang true."

Once these ladies started talking they couldn't stop. One woman, who you will meet in chapter 10, told us that now she tells everybody—men and women—what she has learned since reviewing these chapters. She says when she first mentions incontinence, "They get real quiet and maybe even a little gray in the face. Then, they walk away. But the funny thing is, they often come back later and ask questions."

We hope that after reading this book, you will do the same—actively participate in your treatment, and help yourself and others by asking and answering lots of questions.

CHAPTER 2

URINARY INCONTINENCE

THE BIG PICTURE

"Don't let yourself get used to it."
Claire—urinary incontinence patient

A MORNING AT BLADDER HEALTH CLASS

At a regional hospital a group of women are attending a monthly informational session about bladder control problems. Though they range in age from thirty-two to seventy-four, these women experience the common frustrations and fears that come with urinary incontinence. They are tired of changing out of urine-soaked clothes. They have had it with feeling tethered to the nearest ladies' room. Some are physically exhausted from frequent nighttime rushes to the bathroom; or worse, waking up on wet sheets.

Several are older women who have been dealing with leaky and/or *overactive bladders* for many years. Two are young mothers who had never leaked before becoming pregnant. In this widely mixed group of women few have any idea why they are leaking or what they can do to make it stop.

For unique and very personal reasons, each of these women has decided to take control by seeking treatment. They are here because they will not let urinary incontinence steal their freedom and self-confidence any longer.

The class leader, a nurse from the hospital's continence clinic, begins the session with a video. As the narrator details common difficulties of life without adequate bladder control, many of the women nod in agreement. The women are surprised to learn of the different causes and types of urinary incontinence. They are pleased to find that there are many simple things they can do that will help them regain continence. It could even be as easy as cutting back on *caffeine* and certain spicy foods! "Well, if it helps," one woman sighs, "I could do that."

The film narrator explains the importance of the exercises that help strengthen muscles that support the bladder and uterus. This supportive web is the *pelvic floor*. Several women chuckle as they remember learning about these "Kegels" during their childbirth classes. "Boy, now I wish I had done them!" one woman jokes. They learn about *pessaries* (fig. 2.1), which fit inside the *vagina* and help prevent leaks. The narrator describes physical therapy treatments and explains that certain medications can decrease those frequent bathroom trips. At the mention of surgery some of the women feel a twinge of worry. Most are glad to know surgery can help, but hope other treatments will let them avoid it.

As the video finishes, the nurse says, "Okay, ladies, intermission—the restroom is across the hall." There is more than one sigh of relief. The nurse knows that even twenty minutes can be an uncomfortable wait for some women.

After break, the nurse answers the women's questions. The women want to understand why this is happening to them. They want to hear more about pessaries. They ask if the physical therapy treatments will be painful. They want to know more about dietary and behavior changes that can help improve their continence. They want relief and they want to know how to get started.

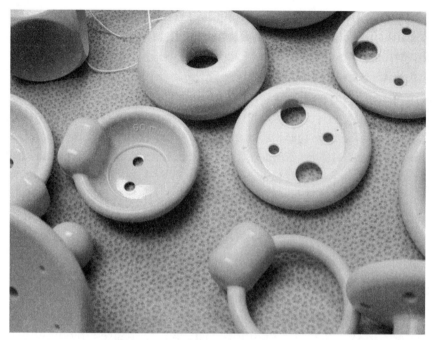

Fig. 2.1. Pessaries fit inside the vagina to help support pelvic organs and improve continence. They are available in many shapes and sizes.

"These are great questions," the nurse says. "I love giving you the good news that pelvic floor muscle exercises combined with behavior changes will help most of you improve your bladder control. For others, medications or surgery may be the answer. But either way, each of you has a great chance for better bladder control!"

THE SILENT EPIDEMIC

The International Continence Society defines urinary incontinence as "a condition where involuntary loss of urine is a social or hygienic problem and is objectively demonstrable." But most women coping with urine leakage will simply say, "Urinary incontinence is just plain embarrassing and uncomfortable." The World Health Organization estimates that in the United States, the number of women who have urinary incontinence ranges from a low value of thirteen million to as many as thirty-three million. This chronic condition affects all age groups, backgrounds, and fitness levels. Women may tolerate bladder control problems for years or even decades, thinking the difficulties are "just part of aging" or that they have no choice. In fact, urinary incontinence has many causes and many treatment options.

In the United States, one in three women over the age of sixty experiences bladder control problems. Of these, 14 percent are incontinent on a daily basis. Although urinary incontinence can occur at any age, it is more common for women to develop urinary incontinence later in their lives. While it is true that *menopause* can cause tissue and muscle changes that may affect bladder control, do not think of urinary incontinence as an incurable consequence of aging. It is a health condition that can be caused by physical changes, and can be treated regardless of age.

Younger women may have urinary incontinence because of childbirth or certain medical problems. Women with jobs that involve frequent heavy lifting can become incontinent from the constant strain on their pelvic organs and related supportive muscles. Women who have muscular problems, back injuries, nerve damage, and urinary tract infections may also develop urinary incontinence. Because it is not usually painful, women may not consider urinary incontinence a serious health condition.

At first, these women may feel that their symptoms are manageable. Most can cope with an occasional leak. But even mild symptoms often become harder to deal with over time. Often, women believe that pads and diapers are the only solution available (fig. 2.2). It is very common that women put off seeking treatment for urinary incontinence until it interferes with their emotional well-being, their overall physical health, and their ability to conduct daily activities.

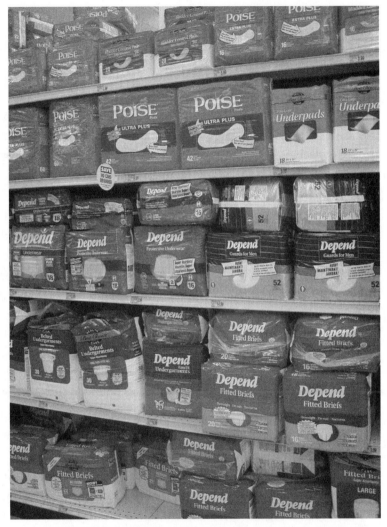

Fig. 2.2. Unfortunately, many incontinent women believe absorbency products are the only option for coping with poor bladder control.

TALKING ABOUT
BLADDER CONTROL PROBLEMS

Some women can talk comfortably about incontinence and its treatments. For many others, the topic is just too embarrassing to discuss—even with a doctor or close family members. It is very helpful for you to talk about your incontinence with friends or trusted relatives. While you may feel uncomfortable at first, you will be surprised how many women you know also share your problem.

Cultural and age-related attitudes about personal or female health issues can affect self-image regarding health and independence. This alone may prevent women from talking openly about urinary incontinence or their own bodies. In addition, women who are uncomfortable touching their private areas, or allowing a doctor to do so, may have difficulty with certain incontinence treatments.

Some women find that exploring why incontinence makes them feel embarrassed helps them overcome their communication barriers. Becoming more familiar with your attitudes about poor bladder control can help you talk more easily with your doctor, your family, or friends about your condition. You can use Worksheet 2C at the end of this chapter as a way to begin reviewing your feelings about urinary incontinence.

Based on what the worksheets in this chapter help you discover about yourself, you may want to begin keeping a reflective journal while you navigate the emotional and physical process of improving your continence. Journal writing is a powerful recovery tool! Looking back at what you have written, even a few days later, will help you to see yourself from a different perspective.

Common misconceptions about bladder control problems, in addition to embarrassment, prevent over half of the women with urinary incontinence from ever seeking help. Congratulations—by reading this book, you are already taking a positive and promising step toward better bladder control! Without a doubt, the more you understand bladder control, the better you can manage your condition. Understanding some general information about the causes and different types of urinary incontinence will help you take steps to improve your continence.

"Gotta Go," "Laugh and Leak," or Both?

Bladder control difficulties can usually be described as the "gotta go" problem or the "laugh and leak" problem. Many women have both types of incontinence. Women with "gotta go" symptoms cope with frequent, sudden, overwhelming urges to urinate, sometimes followed by an unexpected gush of urine. This type of urinary incontinence is called *overactive bladder*. Women who leak when they cough, sneeze, laugh, stand up, or strain to lift something heavy have *stress incontinence*—named for the physical stress, or pressure, the abdominal muscles exert against the bladder with physical activity. You will learn more about each type of incontinence in chapter 3. For now, use Worksheets 2A, 2B, and 2C located at the end of the chapter to begin exploring your urinary incontinence symptoms and the feelings you may have about them. Writing and then reading your responses to worksheet questions will help you to both organize your thoughts and make it easier to talk with your doctor.

THE COSTS OF COPING

Women with urinary incontinence spend a great deal of time, energy, and money coping with their condition. Extra loads of laundry and frequent bathroom stops are time consuming. Bladder control difficulties put women at higher risk for skin and urinary tract infections, and depression. Mad dashes to the bathroom increase risk for falls and fractures. Worry about wetness is exhausting and absorbency products are an endless expense.

Almost always, the practical and emotional cost of coping becomes increasingly difficult as urinary incontinence worsens.

Urinary incontinence is a very expensive condition. According to a study reported in the magazine *OBG Management*, the total costs of urinary incontinence—including things such as laundry, coping with urinary tract infections and depression, absorbency product and clothing purchases, and time lost from work—are at least $26.3 billion per year! This same report states that for each woman over the age of sixty-five, the annual costs of urinary incontinence are $3,565!

What are your costs of coping? Use Worksheet 2B to examine the ways urinary incontinence affects your life.

Daily Life

The challenge of trying to get errands done between bathroom stops and the constant worry about the possibility of embarrassing accidents makes it more practical to stay at home. While absorbency products are helpful leak management tools, they are costly and sometimes bulky.

In addition, taking numerous bathroom breaks at work can bring serious consequences. Regardless of her type of work, every woman has the right to appropriate bathroom breaks. It is a matter of health, not convenience! Once educated about this problem, employers are often willing to accommodate the needs of an incontinent employee. But few women want to discuss such a personal health issue at work. Even with friends or family, incontinent women may feel awkward excusing themselves often to go to the bathroom and may be too embarrassed to explain their condition.

Additionally, urinary incontinence can make driving difficult and using public transportation or walking next to impossible. It can keep women from attending religious services, joining hobby groups, or enjoying travel. Bladder control problems can make a woman feel trapped in her own home.

Emotional

It is no surprise that urinary incontinence affects emotional health—the frustrations women often face when coping with urinary incontinence can cause depression. Women often feel their self-confidence slipping away. Urinary incontinence can put a strain on relationships, too. Friends and loved ones may not understand a woman's reluctance to spend time with them.

Bladder control problems have varied effects on women's sex lives. For some, it is not an issue. But for others, anxiety about wetness or odor, as well as the possibility of leakage, may interfere with intimacy and sexual enjoyment. Regaining or improving continence can have important benefits in this aspect of many women's lives.

Physical

Your overall health may suffer if bladder control problems remain untreated. Incontinent women may use common coping strategies such as limiting physical activity, withdrawing from social settings, decreasing water intake, and waking often at night to rush to the bathroom. However, inactivity, isolation, dehydration, and sleep deprivation may lead to conditions such as obesity and kidney disease, emotional problems, or physical injuries. Incontinent women may also be troubled by skin rashes and frequent urinary tract infections, which are painful and sometimes difficult to treat.

In addition, symptoms of urinary incontinence can be related to having other serious health conditions, including *diabetes*, or neuromuscular disease such as multiple sclerosis. Attempts to tolerate urinary incontinence without seeing a doctor could have other health consequences. To rule out these possibilities, speak to your doctor about your symptoms.

Worsening without Treatment

While many incontinent women notice that their bladder control worsens as they get older, they may not understand that their condition could simply be deteriorating from lack of treatment. You will learn why this happens as our discussion proceeds. But the fact remains that, regardless of cause or severity, bladder control can be improved in nearly all cases.

A HIGHLY TREATABLE CONDITION

Once incontinent patients begin the process of treatment and see how quickly they get some relief, they wish they had sought help much sooner. For example, eight in ten women can improve their bladder control just by making small behavioral changes and by strengthening their pelvic floor muscles! In chapter 4 you will learn more about many simple first-step methods that can help you begin to improve your continence.

TEAMING UP WITH YOUR DOCTOR

It is important to keep in mind that a diagnosis of urinary incontinence takes time and careful evaluation. A diagnosis is a process—not a quick answer. When talking with your doctor about your symptoms, you are providing important clues about the causes and severity of your condition.

If you find that the "first steps" described in chapter 4 do not provide satisfactory results, you and your doctor can explore a number of alternatives. You also need to discuss with your doctor your personal expectations for improved bladder control. Doing this is helpful because incontinence treatment outcomes and women's satisfaction with them can vary widely.

Many doctors who specialize in treating bladder control problems provide care in collaboration with other healthcare specialists such as nurses and physical therapists. In addition to lifestyle changes, behavior modifications, and *pelvic floor exercises*, treatments may include physical therapy, pessaries, prescription medications, as well as major and minor surgeries. How your doctor designs your treatment plan will depend in large part on the services your medical facility offers. In almost all cases, urinary incontinence treatment begins with the least invasive options. Once your doctor evaluates your progress, he or she may suggest adding or using other methods to "fine-tune" your treatment process.

LOOKING AHEAD

It will take time, hard work, and patience but you can improve your bladder control! Regardless of how long you have coped with urinary incontinence, you can learn and relearn effective bladder habits. To meet your individual continence goals, you need to take an active role in your treatment. You also need to be patient and keep an open mind to new ideas and treatment methods during this challenging and rewarding process. The most important part of urinary incontinence treatment is remembering to be as kind to yourself as you would be to a friend having the same problem.

In the next chapter we offer expanded information on urinary and pelvic *anatomy*, how the urinary system works, and why it may stop working properly. This information, including helpful urinary incontinence terminology, will prove useful as you read the remaining chapters and talk with your doctor about bladder control.

WORKSHEETS

Worksheet 2A: My Symptoms

Use this list to identify symptoms you may have and how often you experience them. Use the space provided at the end to describe any other incontinence symptoms you have. This worksheet is also a helpful communication tool—take it with you to your next doctor's appointment.

I leak urine when I cough, laugh, or sneeze: ___ rarely ___ sometimes ___ often	I leak urine because I cannot get to a bathroom quickly enough: ___ rarely ___ sometimes ___ often
I leak urine when I stand up: ___ rarely ___ sometimes ___ often	I leak urine in a sudden gush: ___ rarely ___ sometimes ___ often
I leak urine when I lift something: ___ rarely ___ sometimes ___ often	I leak urine when I hear water running: ___ rarely ___ sometimes ___ often
I leak urine when I am physically active: ___ rarely ___ sometimes ___ often	My urges to urinate feel very strong: ___ rarely ___ sometimes ___ often

I leak urine during sex: ___ rarely ___ sometimes ___ often	My urges to urinate seem frequent: ___ 15 or 20 minutes apart ___ about an hour apart ___ more than 1 hour apart
If you have symptoms in the column above, you may be having stress incontinence.	If you have symptoms in the column above, you may be having overactive bladder (urge incontinence).
If you have symptoms from both columns, you may be having mixed incontinence.	

Other Symptoms and Information:

I have pain with urination:
___ rarely
___ sometimes
___ often

There is blood in my urine:
___ rarely
___ sometimes
___ often

I have a very weak flow of urine:
___ rarely
___ sometimes
___ often

My bladder does not feel like it empties completely:
___ rarely
___ sometimes
___ often

My urinary incontinence symptoms began:
    ___ slowly
    ___ suddenly

I have been having bladder control problems for:
    ___ weeks
    ___ months
    ___ years
    ___ more than 10 years

Other bladder control problems I am having: (list)

_____

_____

_____

_____

_____

_____

_____

_____

Worksheet 2B: My Costs of Coping

Use this worksheet to take an inventory of the ways that bladder control problems may be affecting your lifestyle as well as your emotional and physical health. Mark any statements that apply to your situation. This is another worksheet that can be a helpful communication tool—take it with you to your next doctor's appointment.

Daily Life

I plan my day around bathroom stops:
    ___ rarely
    ___ sometimes
    ___ often
    ___ at all times

I can only go to places that have a restroom:
    ___ rarely
    ___ sometimes
    ___ often
    ___ at all times

Coping with urinary incontinence is distracting:
    ___ rarely
    ___ sometimes
    ___ often
    ___ at all times

I have to change out of urine-soaked clothes:
    ___ rarely
    ___ sometimes
    ___ often
    ___ daily

I use absorbency products:

___ rarely

___ sometimes

___ often

___ at all times

Bladder control problems are affecting my responsibilities:

___ at home

___ at my job

___ other

Emotional

Check all that apply:

___ I feel embarrassed about having this condition

___ I feel anxiety and worry about the possibility of accidents

___ I feel less independent because of incontinence

___ I worry that I will have to live with bladder control problems forever

___ I feel that I need to keep my incontinence a secret from:

    ___ strangers

    ___ coworkers

    ___ friends

    ___ family members

    ___ my spouse or partner

___ Bladder control problems are affecting my relationships:

    ___ at work

    ___ with close friends

    ___ with family

    ___ with my spouse or partner

___ I am missing out on things I enjoy doing because of incontinence

Physical

Check all that apply:

___ I am limiting my physical activity to prevent urine leaks

___ I have skin irritation from urine or absorbency products

___ I avoid drinking water or other liquids

___ I wake at night because of urinary incontinence:

> ___ never
>
> ___ once a night
>
> ___ two to three times a night
>
> ___ more than three times a night

___ I get urinary tract infections:

> ___ rarely
>
> ___ one or two times a year
>
> ___ more than three times a year

___ My urinary accidents are happening more often than they used to

Worksheet 2C: My Feelings about Urinary Incontinence

To explore your attitudes about your condition use the space provided to list some words or thoughts that come to mind for each prompt. You may want to return to these questions after thinking about them a little. It may also be helpful to review this worksheet from time to time during your treatment process.

When I first began having urinary incontinence symptoms, I felt:

_____

_____

Now, having urinary incontinence symptoms feels:

_____

_____

Discussing my condition with friends or family makes me feel:

_____

_____

Discussing my problem with other women who have had urinary incontinence feels:

_____

_____

Discussing my condition with a doctor that I know makes me feel:

_____

_____

Discussing my condition with a doctor that I have not met before makes me feel:

_____

_____

If someone is insensitive about my condition I feel:

_____

_____

Learning about my condition feels:

_____

_____

Learning about the treatment procedures for urinary incontinence feels:

_____

_____

Trying self-help approaches for urinary incontinence makes me feel:

_____

_____

The idea of getting treatment for urinary incontinence feels:

_____

_____

Other feelings I am having about my bladder control problems:

_____

_____

_____

_____

_____

_____

_____

_____

FREQUENTLY ASKED QUESTIONS

1. Will my insurance cover urinary incontinence treatment?

Urinary incontinence is a health condition, and those conditions that have a negative affect on quality of life are usually covered by insurance. Check your policy guidelines carefully or call your insurance provider's customer service department with specific questions. Your doctor's office staff or their billing office may provide you with some general information on this subject.

2. How long will it take before I see improvement?

It will depend on your symptoms and how long you have been having them. As with any other lifestyle or health adjustment you might make, your urinary incontinence treatment results will depend on many factors, one important factor being your level of motivation! With urinary incontinence treatments active patient participation is vital. Other factors include the severity of your condition, your overall health, and your access to the necessary medical treatments.

3. Why do certain foods and drinks affect bladder control?

Foods and beverages contain many different naturally occurring chemical compounds. These chemicals end up in our bloodstream and can affect our organs and tissues in many different ways. For example, the consumption of alcohol and the caffeine found in coffee and in other foods and beverages can temporarily increase the rate of urine production.

CHAPTER 3

GETTING ORIENTED

THE DETAILS OF
URINARY INCONTINENCE

*"I am fifty-six years old and nobody has ever
talked to me about my own body."*
Lisa—at a postoperative interview

"WHY ISN'T MY BLADDER WORKING RIGHT?"

Gina didn't want to have to think about her bladder and she certainly didn't want to have to worry about why it was leaking. She just wanted to know what could be done to fix it. As a healthy and active woman, she was frustrated that her bladder leaks had gotten worse and worse for no apparent reason. Gina knew the situation was beginning to affect her lifestyle, and she was starting to feel self-conscious at work. She could only imagine how bad things would be in a few more years. "Am I going to be homebound and have to rely on others to do my shopping?" she recalls worrying.

When Gina asked her family doctor about the leaks, she learned that poor bladder control is a common problem. Other than that, her doctor did not say or do much except send her home with a pamphlet that described how to do the same "Kegels" or pelvic floor muscle-strengthening exercises that she learned about in her childbirth education sessions.

Back then, the instructor hadn't made it very clear what these exercises would accomplish or why anyone should bother doing them. Now, Gina felt embarrassed asking her doctor these same questions. Besides, she imagined the doctor's explanation would be full of impossible medical terminology. She tried doing the exercises for a few weeks, but couldn't tell if she was doing them right or whether they had made a difference. "Anyway," Gina recalls thinking, "what does squeezing my vagina have to do with keeping my bladder from leaking?"

Recently, she began noticing advertisements on TV and in magazines for overactive bladder medications. "I don't know what is wrong with me," she told her gynecologist during an annual exam, "but I can tell you my problem seems different than what the women in the ads have. I never have that panicky rush to the restroom or any discomfort other than damp or wet underwear several times a day." Several weeks later, as she began urinary incontinence treatment at a women's health center, Gina's first questions for the doctor were, "Why isn't my bladder working right? Why can't it hold urine like it used to?"

GETTING STARTED

Deciding to seek treatment for urinary incontinence is a positive step toward a more comfortable and healthy lifestyle. Many women discover that when they begin looking into bladder control treatment they first find more questions than answers.

Many things can contribute to urinary incontinence, and there are many different approaches to help improve bladder control. It is only natural that patients find themselves facing a steep learning curve as they begin to explore their options. Talking with a doctor about such a private problem can feel uncomfortable, and trying to decode the medical explanations can be frustrating. Just getting accustomed to the doctor's urinary incontinence vocabulary is often a challenge!

Learning a little about the organs and muscles that work together to control your urine flow can be an important first step. Of course, you can regain continence without learning every detail of your urinary system's structure, arrangement, and function. But the more you understand why urinary incontinence happens, the more comfortable you will feel participating in the treatment process.

LEARNING ABOUT URINARY INCONTINENCE

Where is my bladder? How should it work? What is happening when I lose bladder control? You have probably never thought about urinary incontinence in terms of your anatomy and how it is arranged. An easy way to think about your bladder and incontinence is to imagine a water-filled balloon. Using this analogy, your *urethra*, through which the urine passes when you urinate, is represented by the neck of the balloon. The end of your urethra closest to the bladder consists of muscular tissue that contracts tightly to keep urine inside the bladder—just like pinching the balloon neck to prevent air from escaping. This contracting region is the *urethral sphincter*. Now imagine the balloon, neck pointing downward, resting inside your lower abdomen. A hammock-like group of muscles, the *pelvic floor*, supports and correctly positions your pelvic organs. The pelvic floor muscles are important because their ability to maintain the bladder position affects its function and the events that lead to the planned or unplanned urination (fig. 3.1).

Normally, when your bladder is about half full, it contracts and you feel the urge to urinate. When you have this sensation and can choose whether or not to urinate, you know your brain and bladder are working together correctly. This important messaging system is

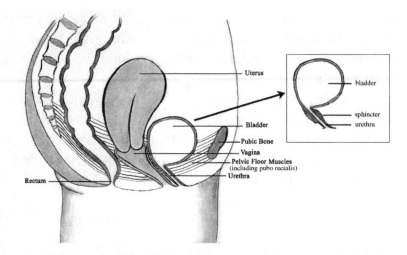

Fig. 3.1. Your pelvic floor is a group of muscles that support your pelvic organs and play an important role in maintaining continence.

a *neurological* connection between your brain and your bladder, something we will call the "brain-bladder" connection.

When you choose to urinate, your brain responds to the *contraction* signal by telling your pelvic floor muscles and the urethral sphincter to relax. This allows urine to flow through the urethra as the bladder contracts. For continence, you need effective coordination between bladder contractions and urethral sphincter relaxations. When something interferes with this coordination, incontinence may occur.

To help you understand how female urinary anatomy works, as well as what happens when things are *not* working correctly, we will first review the normal location and function of key pelvic organs and muscles involved in urine production, storage, and urination.

Urine Production

The kidneys are two fist-sized, bean-shaped organs located just below and behind your lower ribs. These organs continuously filter blood to remove waste substances and water from the bloodstream. As blood trickles through the kidneys' intricate filtering structure, it is cleansed and most of the fluid is returned to the bloodstream. The remaining water and wastes are deposited into the bladder as urine for disposal (fig. 3.2).

Although you may only urinate from time to time throughout the day, your kidneys continuously filter your blood and produce urine. The kidneys produce about five cups of urine each day. Barring extreme dehydration, they make urine even when you do not

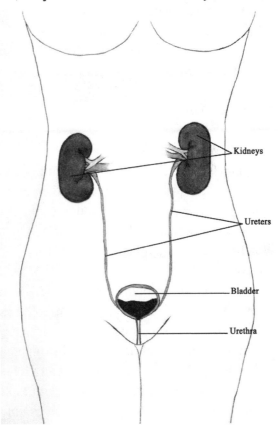

Fig. 3.2. Urine is produced in the kidneys, travels through the ureters to the bladder, and leaves the body through the urethra.

Kidneys

Ureters

Bladder

Urethra

drink enough water and other fluids. That is why limiting your fluid intake is not a healthy way to manage incontinence. In chapter 4 you will learn tips for getting adequate fluids without increasing your symptoms. You will also learn about how dietary fluids can actually help improve your continence by preventing hard stools and *constipation* that increase stress on your pelvic floor muscles.

Your Bladder Has Two Jobs: Storing Urine and Eliminating Urine

Your bladder lies below the kidneys, resting in front of and slightly below the uterus (fig. 3.3). This arrangement is one reason why pregnant women feel the need to urinate often—the growing baby is in essence "sitting" on its mother's bladder. The balloonlike bladder wall is a three-layered muscle, collectively called the *detrusor*, which stretches to allow the bladder to fill. The detrusor muscle contracts, or squeezes, when it is time to urinate.

Storing Urine

Urine travels from the kidneys down and into the bladder through two thin tubes called *ureters*. The ureters open into the bladder on each side, toward its lower half. When certain nerve sensors, called *stretch receptors*, in the bladder walls detect that the bladder is expanding, they signal the brain that it is time to urinate. Usually this happens as the bladder is about half full—with about one cup of urine.

The urethral sphincter, an important region of the bladder neck, prevents urine from leaving the bladder at the wrong time. Although this tissue is not a "true sphincter," many healthcare professionals simply call it a urethral sphincter. This is because, like a sphincter, this tissue closes the urethra by contracting around it.

The urethral sphincter remains tight to keep the upper end of the urethra closed. Recalling our balloon example, you can imagine that

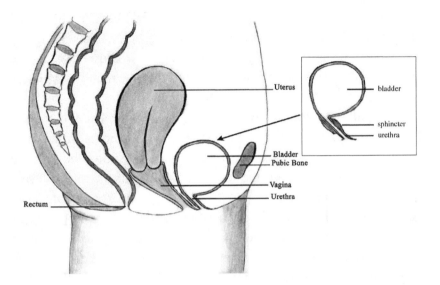

Fig. 3.3. In this simplified diagram of the pelvic organs, note that the upper vaginal wall forms a supportive foundation for the bladder and urethra.

---

if someone applies pressure to the balloon, the urethral sphincter must remain tightly squeezed around the balloon neck to prevent the water from escaping. When your brain sends a signal to the sphincter that it is time to urinate, it relaxes as part of the process that allows urine to pass through the urethra and out of the body.

Eliminating Urine

Most women feel the urge to urinate about every three hours. The bladder begins contracting long before it is completely full. It is usually possible to ignore urge sensations until it is convenient to get to the bathroom. Often, when you ignore these signals, the urgency feelings fade temporarily and return with greater force a short time later.

When you urinate, urine travels from the bladder out of the body through a tube called the urethra. The urethra lies alongside the muscle walls of the *vagina* and opens just above the vaginal opening. The *rectum* and its opening, the *anus*, are positioned behind the vagina.

Normally, the process of urination, or *voiding*, has three steps. First, the bladder contracts in response to becoming filled with urine. Then, if you choose to urinate, impulses along the *nervous system* pathways signal the urethral sphincter to relax. These impulses also trigger relaxation of the pelvic floor. You urinate when your bladder contracts and your urethra and pelvic floor are relaxed.

However, there are some variations on this typical urination process. You may urinate, sometimes or always, by bearing down as you do during a bowel movement. Some women do this when they are in a hurry. This bearing down, or what is called a *Valsalva maneuver*, causes your *diaphragm* and abdominal muscles to contract. This creates pressure against the bladder—causing it to expel urine faster. In another variation, with or without realizing it, you may relax your pelvic floor muscles first. When your pelvic floor muscles relax, the urethra will relax as well because these regions share a nervous system pathway called a *reflex arc*. Once the urethral sphincter relaxes, you urinate.

Your Abdominal Organ Support Structure

As you have learned, a hammock-like foundation of muscles and soft tissue connections called the pelvic floor supports your urinary and abdominal organs. These layers of muscle, anchored on the pelvic bones, help keep the abdominal organs positioned correctly within the bowl formed by your pelvis. The urethra, vagina, and rectum pass between the muscles and connective tissues of the pelvic floor. Even though the pelvic floor muscles, urethral sphincter, and urethra are loosely connected individual tissues, they work together to keep urine within the bladder until brain signals tell you it is time to urinate (fig. 3.1).

TYPES OF URINARY INCONTINENCE

Now that you have a better sense of urinary anatomy you can more easily understand the four most common types of urinary incontinence, the factors that contribute to them, and the treatments available for each type.

There are four common types of urinary incontinence:

1. Overactive bladder or urge incontinence ("gotta go")
2. Stress incontinence ("laugh and leak")
3. Mixed incontinence (a combination of overactive bladder and stress incontinence)
4. Overflow incontinence (rare)

A Quick Look at Urinary Incontinence Types

The main difference between overactive bladder and stress incontinence is the involvement of the detrusor muscle. In overactive bladder, detrusor muscle activity is a key factor because the detrusor muscle contracts when it should not. However, in stress incontinence, the detrusor is passive, or quiet, meaning that detrusor muscle activity itself is not the direct cause of urine loss. The stress on the bladder literally forces the urethral sphincter to open and allows urine to pass, as when a laugh or a sneeze results in unexpected urination.

An important difference between symptoms of overactive bladder and stress incontinence is the way urine is lost. Overactive bladder usually causes sudden overwhelming urges to urinate, often followed by an uncontrollable loss of a large amount of urine. The urge sensation that accompanies overactive bladder is often impossible to suppress. Overactive bladder is more common in older women.

In comparison, stress incontinence usually causes small spurts of urine to escape when you laugh, cough, sneeze, stand up, or lift something. Stress incontinence may also cause frequent urine dribbling, with or without additional spurts that result from coughing or sneezing. Stress incontinence is more common in younger women. Women with mixed incontinence have a combination of both stress and urge symptoms.

It is not unusual for women to experience one or both types of urinary incontinence for a short period, perhaps a few weeks, at some point in their lives. Common reasons for short-term urinary incontinence include pregnancy and delivery of a baby, urinary tract infections, certain medications, or recovery from abdominal surgery. It is especially important for women who have urinary incontinence after childbirth to learn how to do pelvic floor exercises and begin doing them daily. Since pelvic floor exercises are cost-free and easy to perform, making them a part of your normal routine makes sense. Chapter 4 provides easy-to-follow instructions to help you learn how to do pelvic floor muscle exercises most effectively.

Overflow incontinence is a more rare fourth type of urinary incontinence. With this condition the bladder never completely empties or does not signal the urge to urinate even when it is very full. Overflow incontinence may be caused by an obstruction that prevents urine from flowing freely through the urethra. Such an obstruction can occur when the pelvic organs shift out of their normal position because of poor pelvic organ support. Other causes include nerve or tissue damage to the spinal cord or to the detrusor muscle. Diabetes can also cause nerve or tissue damage that prevents the bladder from emptying completely. Women with overflow incontinence often constantly dribble urine. Some also have stress or urge symptoms. Some may experience discomfort from having an overfilled bladder that they cannot effectively empty. Other health problems that may occur as a result of urine retention include bladder infections, and in extreme cases, kidney damage when urine backs up into the kidneys.

OVERACTIVE BLADDER: THE DETAILS

An overactive detrusor muscle, or bladder wall, causes overactive bladder symptoms. The entire urinary system, including the detrusor muscle, is controlled by the nervous system. Recall that your brain-bladder connection is actually nervous system signals that run between your brain and bladder. Simply put, overactive bladder results from a pattern of miscommunication between your brain and your bladder. This causes the muscles inside the wall of the bladder to contract inappropriately—too forcefully, too often, or both! These urges can be overwhelmingly strong even though the bladder may not be full. Women with overactive bladder often cannot suppress or ignore such abnormally strong urge sensations.

The source of the miscommunication is often caused by signals that arise in the detrusor muscle itself. On the other hand, sometimes it is because of a problem in the nerve pathways that send signals between the brain and bladder. But either way, the unfortunate result is that you do not always get to choose when you urinate.

Such miscommunication can be caused by damage to the nervous system from stroke, spinal cord injury, back problems, multiple sclerosis, diabetes, Parkinson's disease, or certain medications. Spicy or acidic foods, alcohol, caffeine, and nicotine can also contribute in differing ways to overactive bladder symptoms. A simple bladder or urinary tract infection, kidney stones, a pelvic exam, or sexual intercourse can also cause these symptoms. It is not always possible to determine the cause of overactive bladder.

Types of Overactive Bladder

Overactive bladder can fall under the following four headings:

1. Urinary urgency
2. Urinary frequency
3. Both urinary urgency and frequency
4. Nocturia (overactive bladder symptoms at night)

Women with urinary urgency have sudden and extremely strong urges to urinate. When such sensations happen, these women can only think of getting to the restroom in time, and they may need to drop whatever they are doing to do so.

Urinary frequency is defined as feeling the need to urinate more than eight to ten times in a twenty-four-hour period. Women with this condition are faced with unnecessary, uncomfortable, and distracting urge symptoms. It is very common for women to have overactive bladder with both urgency and frequency.

In many cases, overactive bladder symptoms continue through the night. This condition is called *nocturia*. Waking up once a night to go to the bathroom is not considered abnormal, but women with overactive bladder may wake up twice or even several times a night because they feel the need to urinate. Or, they may wake up too late and find themselves in a urine-soaked bed. Wetting yourself while sleeping is called *nocturnal enuresis*. Chapter 4 provides many useful dietary, fluid intake, and medication management tips to help minimize accidents or trips to the bathroom during the day and night.

You may be surprised to learn that some women who have urgency, frequency, and nocturia do not usually leak urine. Overactive bladder without leaks is called *"dry" overactive bladder*. Overactive bladder with leaks is called *"wet" overactive bladder*. Many factors can affect whether or not overactive bladder is accompanied by leaks. But with or without leaks, overactive bladder and the frequent feeling that one "has to go" can have a profound effect on women's freedom, peace of mind, and ability to sleep well.

The Brain-Bladder Connection and Overactive Bladder

So why *does* the detrusor muscle become overactive? What causes brain-bladder connection miscommunication? As the bladder fills, signals that originate from the stretch receptors in your detrusor muscle travel from your bladder to your brain. Your brain responds by sending signals to the bladder, either telling the detrusor to contract or not to contract because there is no bathroom handy. Up to a point, you can override or ignore these signals when you choose not to urinate.

With overactive bladder, the stretch receptors may develop a pattern of sending overly frequent "time to urinate" signals that your brain may not be able to stop. While the stretch receptors would normally signal "time to urinate" when the bladder is about half filled, they may inappropriately send these signals even when your bladder is only slightly filled. Overactive bladder symptoms may also result from the brain sending strong and/or frequent contraction signals to the detrusor without having received any feedback from the stretch receptors (fig. 3.4).

Many women with overactive bladder have "triggers" that initiate or aggravate this difficult cycle and stimulate the bladder to empty suddenly. Triggers may include thinking about urinating, unlocking the door when arriving at home, entering the bathroom, seeing a toilet, hearing running water, or even feeling anxious. Anyone who has had to dance at the door while trying to unlock it knows what these feelings are like!

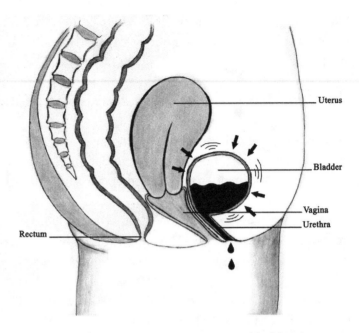

Fig. 3.4. Women with overactive bladder have frequent strong "time to urinate" signals generated by the stretch receptors in the bladder. Leaking occurs when your brain cannot suppress these contractions.

STRESS INCONTINENCE: THE DETAILS

Women with stress incontinence often leak urine when they cough, sneeze, laugh, stand up, or strain to lift something heavy. This symptom happens because abdominal pressure, or stress, increases with these and other physical actions. Abdominal stress can cause urine to leak if the urethral sphincter cannot contract strongly enough to prevent urine flow.

To feel your abdominal muscles at work, lie down on the floor and put your hands over your stomach. Now cough. You should feel a downward pressure of your stomach muscles. This strong pressure *on* your bladder, rather than pressure created *by* your bladder, is what can cause you to leak urine.

Stress incontinence happens when the abdominal pressure is greater than what the urethral sphincter can withstand. This situation may occur because the urethral sphincter is weak or because pelvic floor muscles are sagging. As you will learn later in this chapter, pelvic floor muscles that become weakened or stretched may allow the bladder and urethra to fall out of position, affecting the urethra's ability to hold urine in.

Things that can lead to or aggravate stress incontinence include physical damage from childbirth and increases in abdominal pressure caused by obesity, coughing, heavy lifting, and chronic constipation. Other stress incontinence factors include changes in muscle tone resulting from age-related declines in hormones, the nerve damage caused by diabetes, and the side effects associated with certain medications.

Your Urethra's Role in Stress Incontinence

The key to understanding stress incontinence is to understand your urethra's role in the balance of pressures. There are two important factors in stress incontinence that involve the urethra:

1. Urethral Pressure—the amount of contraction pressure the urethra can maintain
2. Urethral Mobility—the amount the urethra moves when abdominal pressure increases

Urethral pressure helps counteract the effect of abdominal pressure against the bladder. Urethral pressure is defined in varying degrees of "low pressure," "normal pressure," and every point in between.

Urethral mobility is a change in the angle and position of your urethra when a cough or sneeze increases the abdominal pressure.

Urethra mobility is important because if the urethra shifts with an increase in abdominal pressure, it may not be able to maintain the pressure needed to prevent urine loss.

Urethral pressure and urethral mobility are individual but inter-related factors. It is their *combined* effect that determines the severity of a woman's stress incontinence.

Urethra Pressure

The simple truth about stress incontinence is that when the pressure against the bladder exceeds the pressure the urethra is capable of withstanding, you will leak. In turn, you will remain dry as long as your urethra has a higher pressure than any pressure inside your bladder (fig. 3.5).

A urethra that has walls with sufficiently strong muscle tone can stay squeezed closed effectively. A urethra with poor muscle tone is called a low-pressure urethra, which may leak with any increase in abdominal pressure, such as the pressure caused when you stand up, walk up stairs, or pick up a jug of milk. A woman's overall fitness level is not related to her urethra muscle tone. Reasons women may have a low-pressure urethra can include genetics, tissue changes that come with age, or side effects from previous surgeries. Radiation therapy or the tissue changes that medical conditions such as diabetes cause can also lead to this condition.

Urethra Mobility

The mobility, or degree of movement, your urethra has can also affect its ability to stay squeezed tightly enough to prevent stress incontinence leaks. It is important to understand that the bladder and urethra are not oriented vertically. The urethra extends down, and slightly forward, from the bladder neck. Because of this orientation, and because the urethra rests on the vagina, the urethra may shift position if the pelvic floor does not keep the vagina properly

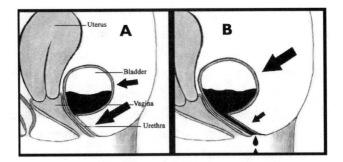

Fig. 3.5. You will leak when bladder pressure is greater than urethral pressure. In figure 3.5a, urethral pressure is greater than bladder pressure, as represented by the large and small arrows, therefore you will not leak. In figure 3.5b, bladder pressure is greater than urethral pressure, and therefore you will leak.

positioned when your abdominal pressure increases as you cough, sneeze, or lift something (fig. 3.5).

Why does it matter if the urethra is mobile? It matters because when the urethra shifts position, the abdominal pressure is then distributed unequally to the bladder and urethra. When the urethra moves, the result is that greater pressure is applied to the bladder than to the urethra. Recall that when pressure on the bladder exceeds pressure on the urethra, you will leak.

Your Pelvic Floor and Stress Incontinence

You now know that stress incontinence is associated with muscles other than the detrusor itself. You have also learned that your pelvic floor condition and the position of your bladder neck and urethra affects proper bladder function. You also understand that strong pelvic floor muscles help increase urethral pressure and minimize urethral mobility.

So, what causes the pelvic floor muscles to stretch and possibly even separate? What can be done to get things back to normal?

The pelvic floor muscles, like all muscles and soft tissue connections in your body, lose their ability to function properly when they are damaged or weakened. There are many reasons pelvic floor muscles lose their ability to adequately support your abdominal organs. Some of these reasons include having undergone pelvic surgery, genetics, childbirth, heavy lifting, frequent straining with constipation, chronic coughing, and obesity. Many clinicians believe the hormonal changes that come with aging can also lead to sagging pelvic floor muscles and a weakened urethral sphincter. This is because decreases in *estrogen* often change women's tissue elasticity and muscle tone.

Childbirth can cause permanent damage to the pelvic muscles or cause their connection points on the pelvic bones to detach. Severe pressure on the pelvic muscles can cause irreversible muscle tissue loss (*atrophy*) by injuring the nerves that stimulate muscle contraction or by causing direct injury to the muscle from pressure. Even the ongoing pressure caused by obesity or chronic coughing can strain pelvic floor muscle connections. Muscles cannot contract effectively when they are weak, damaged, or are not solidly attached to bones.

You will recall that when the pelvic floor muscles and connective tissue are in their correct positions and support the bladder correctly, the bladder neck and urethra can remain as tightly closed as possible. But when pelvic floor muscles sag, the orientation of the bladder and urethra changes. This situation adversely affects the balance of pressures between the bladder and urethra and can cause leaking.

The Sneeze and Cough Trick

Think about this: if you tend to leak a little when you sneeze or cough, you may have noticed something different when you have had the "advance notice" of a gradually building sneeze. Without realizing why, many women have learned the trick of preventing leaks by "preparing" for sneezes and coughs by tensing their pelvic area muscles or crossing their legs tightly just before the sneeze. Sometimes these actions will minimize or prevent the leak because you, without realizing it, have contracted your pelvic floor muscles.

Although this scenario is not always a practical solution to managing urinary incontinence, it can help you better understand the role your pelvic floor plays in bladder control. Without knowing it, when you know a sneeze is about to occur, you instinctively "hold in" your pelvic area, thus preventing leaks by partially contracting your pelvic floor and urethra. This contraction is similar to the action you will use when you do pelvic floor muscle exercises. The pelvic floor muscle tension you create for yourself briefly hoists your pelvic floor up into proper position and stabilizes the position of your urethra.

Similarly, crossing your legs can help prevent or minimize loss of urine. This works in the short term because it creates counter-pressure that helps your urethral sphincter resist the force of urine being pushed out by the abdominal pressure of a sneeze or cough.

FINDING SOLUTIONS

If you have urinary incontinence, you may not care as much *why* it is happening—you just want it to stop. Now that you are better acquainted with how your urinary system is arranged and how it works, you are better prepared to take the next steps in the process of regaining continence. The knowledge you have gained about the causes and symptoms of different types of urinary incontinence can help you focus on the "first steps" presented in chapter 4, which may help you the most. As you incorporate these first steps into your daily life, you will likely be surprised at the positive difference they can make. If you find that your first steps do not provide enough relief, you will gain some basic information that can help you talk with your *healthcare provider* more effectively about your condition and the treatment options available.

FREQUENTLY ASKED QUESTIONS

1. If my doctor tells me I have a mobile urethra, does that mean I will need to have surgery to keep it from moving too much?

No, many women have a mobile urethra without any symptoms of incontinence. Surgery for stress urinary incontinence is only indicated when incontinence is bothersome to you.

2. If I exercise and walk more, will my pelvic floor get stronger?

No, although staying active is beneficial to your overall health, you need to strengthen the muscles of the pelvic floor with special exercises. In chapter 4 you will learn how to do pelvic floor exercises.

3. Did jogging make my pelvic floor sag?

Jogging and other physical fitness activities improve overall health for most women without causing pelvic floor muscles to sag. Other activities, such as heavy weight lifting, put excessive strain on pelvic floor muscles and can be associated with loss of bladder control. There are not always clear answers to why a woman's pelvic floor muscles sag. As part of your treatment process, your doctor will help you determine if there are specific activities you need to stop and/or others you should continue.

4. If my bladder is a muscle and it is overactive, is there a medicine that will just relax it and solve the problem?

Medicines can help with the problem of overactive bladder, and for many patients, they may be the solution. However, studies have shown that behavior modification approaches are more effective than medications; they are cheaper and free of side effects. Combinations of medicines with behavioral therapy may have even better results.

5. I never used to have these terrible urges to go to the bathroom all the time, now I do. What changed?

Most women's overactive bladder condition is "idiopathic," meaning that we don't really ever fully understand what has caused it. Fortunately, overactive bladder can be treated even when your doctor has no clear indication why the condition has developed.

6. What is the difference between a ureter and a urethra?

The ureters drain the kidneys, releasing newly formed urine into the bladder for storage. The urethra drains the bladder, releasing urine out of the body.

7. When I push to have a bowel movement, urine spurts out. Is this urinary incontinence?

No. Many women have bowel movements and urinate at the same time.

8. Even though I am almost to the bathroom door, my bladder just lets go! Why can't I hold it just a few seconds longer?

This frustrating situation happens because the brain-bladder connection is not working effectively. Even without realizing it, just anticipating approaching relief of reaching the toilet can distract your brain from suppressing strong bladder contractions. To counter this, try performing a pelvic floor exercise as you approach the bathroom. Contracting the pelvic floor muscles actually relaxes the bladder because of a nervous system reflex arc, described earlier, that the pelvic floor muscles and the bladder share.

9. I leaked a lot in the first months after my second baby was born. Does this mean I will be incontinent when I am older?

This is a possibility. Therefore, it is especially important for women who have had urinary incontinence in the months after childbirth to perform pelvic floor exercises daily to improve their chances for continence in the future.

10. I have diabetes. How does having diabetes affect bladder control?

Diabetes is a complex disease. Having elevated blood sugar causes water to move from other parts of your body into your blood. Eventually this results in the production of large amounts of urine, dehydration, and thirst. Making this much urine is difficult for anyone to manage. However, for women who have additional bladder-related problems, having uncontrolled diabetes can cause a loss of continence.

For reasons that are not clearly understood, diabetes causes widespread bodily damage. Diabetes adversely affects the heart, the veins, and arteries that carry blood throughout the body. Poor blood circulation impairs the ability of nerves, muscles, and all other organs to work properly.

You may have heard of people who have diabetes losing feeling in their feet and hands. The nerve damage that causes loss of sensation there can also affect the nerves that stimulate bladder and pelvic muscle contractions. Certain diagnostic tests you will learn about in chapter 6 can help determine if nerve damage is making bladder control difficult.

CHAPTER 4

FIRST STEPS

TRY THESE AT HOME

"Glory be—they keep you from leaking and nobody knows you are wearing them."

Marina—an incontinence patient
who uses absorbency products

SMALL CHANGES CAN MAKE A BIG DIFFERENCE!

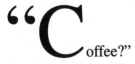

"**C**offee?"

"None for me, but thanks anyway."

You might be surprised to find that some very simple lifestyle changes can greatly reduce and sometimes even eliminate urgency and leaking. Certainly Frances, a textbook editor, was very pleased when her doctor helped her make this discovery.

"I was working on a huge project when my bladder started to boss me around. It made concentrating on my editing impossible because I never knew when I would have to make a mad dash to the bathroom. After a while, it seemed as though that was all I thought about."

Finally, Frances went to see her doctor. Fully prepared to hear that she needed an operation, she was more than surprised when her doctor told her to keep a voiding diary and record things such as the types and amounts of beverages she drank. At first she thought this was total foolishness and that her doctor was giving her distracting busy work.

"I told him I didn't have time for this nonsense. In addition to my job, I was also taking care of my mother as well as trying to have a family life, too. I told him I needed to keep a voiding diary like I needed a 'hole in my head.'"

However, after her doctor told her that substances in certain foods can irritate the bladder and cause urgency, she decided to give the voiding diary an honest try. Doing this revealed two interesting things. First, most of her urgency incidents came shortly after drinking coffee and second—she drank a lot of coffee!

"I guess I needed the voiding diary to notice there was actually a pattern to my bathroom trips. I also didn't realize how much coffee I was drinking at work. I guess I was using the coffee pot down the hall as an excuse to get away from my desk for a few minutes."

To get the relief she needed, Frances made a few simple changes. Rather than using coffee breaks as a way to get away from her desk, she developed the habit of taking a noontime walk. She also found that she didn't need to stop drinking coffee entirely. Limiting herself to a single cup at breakfast or dinner—though even this still sometimes caused problems—conveniently allowed her to manage urgency at home.

BEGINNING YOUR JOURNEY

In this chapter, you will learn some alternative ways to control incontinence and improve continence. The methods are simple and low-technology solutions that you can do at home. However, they are not "quick fixes." All of these first-step methods take patience, persistence, and time. Some of them, such as modifications in dietary and smoking habits, require permanent lifestyle changes.

Regaining continence is your goal. Like Frances, it is also important for you to consider the value of improved or managed continence. Sometimes doing things like pelvic floor exercises, eating more fruit, and drinking more water are helpful. Your symptoms, even though not eliminated, may become controllable and you can return to your active lifestyle. This outcome may not be as good as you had hoped. But you may decide that managing incontinence is a "good enough" solution.

As you will soon learn, keeping a voiding diary is your most important "first step" for treating overactive bladder symptoms. Doing so will help you discover voiding patterns and incontinence triggers. Later, if you decide to seek medical care, this information will help your physician evaluate your situation.

DIARIES AND SELF-REFLECTION

Many people keep a daily diary. Doing this type of reflective writing is a relaxing and therapeutic way to sort out events. Later, taking the time to review diary writings helps them understand the effect that interpersonal, lifestyle, and behavioral influences have on their daily life.

Keeping a voiding diary, such as the one provided in Worksheet 4A at the end of this chapter, will help you associate incidents of leaking and urgency to your typical bathroom habits, patterns of physical activities, and the usual beverages you consume. By doing this simple exercise you might discover a relationship between your morning caffeinated coffee and the urgency and leaking that you experience shortly thereafter. It is also important to consider the other first-step bladder control methods offered in table 4.1.

Table 4.1.
First Steps Guide: Which Method Helps Which Problem?

First-Step Method	Overactive Bladder	Stress Incontinence
Voiding Diary	Yes	Yes
Pelvic Floor Exercises	Yes	Yes
Scheduled Urination Exercises	Yes	No
Diet	Yes	Yes
Drinking Enough Water	Yes	Yes
Fluid and Drug Management	Yes	Yes
Fiber Intake	No	Yes
Lose Weight	No	Yes
Stop Smoking	Yes	Yes

As you can see, most of these first steps help women with both overactive bladder and stress incontinence!

STRENGTHENING YOUR PELVIC FLOOR

Strong pelvic floor muscles help women control urine flow. Pregnancy and childbirth, excess weight, and chronic coughing are some life cycle and lifestyle events that weaken the pelvic floor muscles. Nearly every woman has some of the risk factors associated with pelvic floor weakening. Therefore, many clinicians believe all women, beginning in their teenage years, should regularly perform *pelvic floor exercises.*

Fortunately, pelvic floor weakness does not have to be a permanent condition. Pelvic floor exercises, just like taking a daily walk to make the heart muscle beat more efficiently, can improve pelvic floor strength. However, unlike heart muscle contractions, pelvic floor contractions are voluntary movements that you control. Sometimes, if the pelvic floor muscles are very weak, women have to relearn how to flex them.

To exercise pelvic floor muscles, you need to "squeeze" your vagina as though you are trying to stop urine flow. Some health professionals tell patients to "try pushing your vagina up toward your belly button." This is the same squeeze that pushes a tampon into a more comfortable position. Place your finger inside your vagina. If you feel upward pressure when you squeeze, you are flexing the right muscles.

The trick is to keep other nearby muscles relaxed as you do your pelvic floor exercises. When you squeeze your pelvic floor muscles, your thigh, buttock, and stomach muscles should remain still. Contracting these larger muscle groups when you do your pelvic floor exercises makes it difficult to focus on your pelvic floor muscles. For many women, isolating and flexing the pelvic floor muscle group takes practice!

You can do pelvic floor exercises in nearly any position. However, gravity makes doing them when standing up more difficult. Many women prefer doing pelvic floor exercises while lying on their back with their knees bent. For a more challenging pelvic floor workout, consider doing these exercises while sitting in a chair or standing.

Although the squeeze motion is just like the one used to stop urine flow in midstream, *never do pelvic floor exercises when urinating*. Doing this may contribute to bladder-brain miscommunication and make it difficult to empty your bladder normally.

Whether you decide to lie on your back, sit, or stand, it is important to relax and to breathe normally. Do not hold your breath while doing your pelvic floor exercises.

There are three different ways of doing these exercises. "Quick flicks" is when you quickly contract your pelvic floor muscles, hold for one second, and then relax for one second. Doing "quick flicks" is also a good way to suppress urge feelings—making it easier to make it to the bathroom on time. "Contract and release" is when you tighten your pelvic floor muscles, hold the squeeze for three to four seconds, and then relax.

Another pelvic floor exercise pattern is "the elevator." This is when you partially tighten your pelvic floor muscles, hold for one to two seconds, tighten more, hold for one to two seconds, and then increase the tightness level one more time. However, rather than quickly releasing the squeeze, let go of the pressure one notch at a time. Without question, doing this takes practice! Pictorial representations of the three pelvic floor exercise patterns in figure 4.1 will help you visualize what you need to do.

Pelvic floor exercises can be done anywhere. You can do them at home, sitting at your desk at work, standing in grocery store lines, or even while waiting at traffic lights. Some women find it helpful to listen to music when they do their exercises. Whatever you decide, the most important thing is *to do them regularly*. Use Worksheet 4B located at the end of this chapter to track your pelvic floor exercise progress.

Aim for two five-minute pelvic floor exercise sessions each day. At first, it will be difficult to do these exercises for the full five minutes. Do not get discouraged. Soon, muscle tone will improve and you will be able to reach your goal. Then, when four-second intervals become easy, consider squeezing and relaxing for eight-second intervals!

It takes three to six weeks before most women notice an improvement. Research shows that performing pelvic floor exercises for at least three months can reduce and sometimes even eliminate incontinence problems in nearly 60 to 80 percent of women. Although three months sounds like a long time, it is a worthwhile investment. Pelvic floor exercises, especially when performed in combination with the other "first step" methods discussed in this chapter, are a risk-free and cost-free way to reduce urgency and stress incontinence symptoms and to improve continence.

RETRAINING YOUR BLADDER

Brain-bladder miscommunication produces the strong and inappropriately frequent bladder muscle contractions that cause overactive

Fig. 4.1. Pictorial representation of the three pelvic floor exercise patterns.

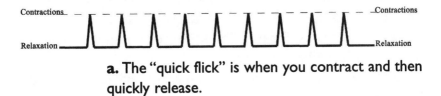

a. The "quick flick" is when you contract and then quickly release.

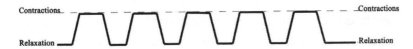

b. The "contract and release" is when you contract and hold the squeeze for three to four seconds and then release.

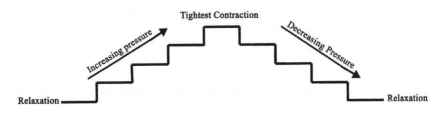

c. The "elevator" is when, in a step-wise fashion, you gradually increase and decrease the squeeze pressure.

---

bladder symptoms. Even though your bladder may not be full, these contractions produce overwhelming and difficult-to-control urination urges.

Women who have strong bladder urges worry and feel anxious about getting to the bathroom in time. Having urge incontinence makes it difficult to work, relax, and participate in daily activities.

Many women, in their efforts to avoid accidents, go to the bathroom more often. Making extra "just in case" trips may worsen overactive bladder problems by confusing normal bladder-brain communication. Doing this may cause the brain to lose the ability to reduce bladder urges. These women have to cope with bladder urges as frequently as every thirty minutes. Some clinicians believe that women may develop urge incontinence as a result of trying to avoid stress incontinence leaks.

Scheduled urination exercise is a process where the clock, rather than bladder urges, determines when you go to the bathroom. Although this may sound a little rigorous, remember you are already making frequent bathroom trips. Scheduling bathroom trips modifies what you are already doing to improve your situation. Many clinicians call scheduled urination "bladder drills" or "timed voidings."

One of the scheduled urination exercise goals is to reduce the amount of time that urination, bathrooms, and accidents dominate your thoughts and interfere with your daily activities. Therefore, it is important to use a timing device such as a kitchen timer or an alarm clock to schedule bathroom visits.

Scheduled urination exercises will help you gradually:

- Increase the amount of urine your bladder can hold before you feel the urge to urinate
- Increase the time between emptying your bladder to once every two to four hours
- Decrease feelings of urgency
- Decrease urine leakage

Plan on beginning your scheduled urination program when you can be home or reliably near a bathroom for a few days. It is also helpful to wear clothes that are easy to remove to reduce the stress of getting to the toilet in time.

Use Worksheet 4C to make a urination schedule that fits your personal needs. The following will give you some ideas about how to design your bladder-retraining program.

- Days 1–3: After awakening, empty your bladder every hour on the hour. Do this even if you do not feel urination urges. Remember to consume the equivalent of six to eight glasses of fluid per day. During the night go to the bathroom only if you waken and find it necessary. If you have the urge to go when it is not yet your scheduled time, DO NOT GO! Keeping to the schedule is what retrains your bladder. If, at first, you cannot wait one hour, it is okay to begin with fifteen- or thirty-minute intervals.
- Days 4–6: Increase the time between emptying your bladder to once every 1½ hours. Follow the above fluid intake and night instructions.
- Days 7–9: Increase the time between emptying your bladder to once every two hours. Follow the above fluid intake and night instructions.
- Days 10–12: Increase the time between emptying your bladder to once every 2½ hours. Follow the above fluid intake and night instructions.
- Days 12 and ongoing: Increase the time between emptying your bladder to once every three to four hours. Continue the above fluid intake and night instructions.

Do keep in mind that the above schedule may not be appropriate for you. Some women may need to begin their bladder-retraining program by emptying their bladder more frequently. It is also permissible to lengthen or even shorten the number of days that you stay at each retraining increment. You are the best judge of how quickly you can advance to the next step.

Even with a schedule, you will still have strong urination urges. The following techniques help many women overcome these strong feelings, extend the time between voidings, and prevent accidents.

- Stay away from voiding triggers such as dripping water or even dressing in the bathroom

- Do several "quick flick" pelvic floor exercise movements before making your way to the bathroom
- Take a deep breath, exhale, and focus on relaxing other muscle groups such as your neck and shoulders
- Change position—either sit down or stand up until the urge passes
- Focus your attention on another activity such as reading or television
- And because it is easier to control the "urge feeling" when you are still, *slowly* make your way to the bathroom

Eventually, when you have reestablished healthy bladder-brain communication, these inappropriate urges will subside and may even disappear. In fact, a study of 197 women at the University of Alabama showed that completing an eight-week scheduled urination program reduces symptoms in eight out of every ten women who have urge incontinence, and worked better than medicines or placebo.

Many women, when they first begin their bladder-retraining program, will have leaks and maybe even a few accidents. If this should happen to you—do not give up. Just like learning how to ride a bicycle, everybody falls a few times before getting the hang of it. Using absorbency products, just like training wheels, will help make the retraining process less frustrating. You can relax and not feel that you have to rush to the bathroom to prevent having an accident when you have absorbency protection. In fact, because rushing makes it even more difficult to control urges, running to the bathroom increases the likelihood of losing bladder control!

Without question, completing your scheduled urination exercise program takes dedication. Many women say that if you can get through the first three days, the rest is comparatively easy. Those who complete their program glow about accomplishments that range from greatly improving their urge incontinence symptoms to actually regaining continence!

DIET

What you eat is one of many lifestyle factors that can interfere with good bladder control. People who do not have enough *fiber* and water in their diet produce hard dry stools that are difficult to pass. This is *constipation*. Pushing to have a bowel movement puts extra pressure on your urethral sphincter and pelvic floor muscles. Over time this may worsen or even cause stress incontinence.

In addition to constipation, there are other links between bowel and bladder function that medical researchers currently do not completely understand. However, most researchers and clinicians agree that it is difficult for your bladder to function optimally when your bowels are not working well.

While increasing the amount of fiber in your diet can improve continence, consumption of certain foods can actually contribute to incontinence. Some women find that eating spicy foods or citrus fruit and drinking beverages containing caffeine or artificial sweeteners make bladder control problems more difficult.

While dietary changes do not always improve continence, many women do report improved bladder control. For many, this means their incontinence is manageable and does not require more invasive treatment strategies.

Water In—Water Out

It is important to consume the equivalent of six to eight glasses of water each day to help prevent constipation and the pressure bearing down puts on the bladder and *pelvic floor* muscles. While this sounds like a lot to drink, it includes the fluid contained in other beverages and in moist or wet foods. Looking at the color of your urine will tell if you are getting enough liquid in your diet. Light yellow or "straw-colored" urine is your goal. Dark yellow urine means you need to drink more. If your urine is nearly colorless, this means you may be consuming too much fluid.

The weather and your physical activity can influence how much water you need to make straw-colored urine. For example, during the hot summer months sweating and the resulting water loss means that you may need to drink more than you might during the cooler seasons.

Keep in mind that taking vitamins and other medications can affect urine color. Taking a daily multivitamin pill and vitamin B and carotene supplements produces bright yellow urine. Using certain laxatives can cause you to produce bright yellow or even orange urine. Because taking these medications may make it difficult for you to tell if you are really drinking enough water, you need to measure your fluid intake.

Managing Your Fluid Intake

Drinking six to eight cups of liquid each day may sound a little self-defeating to women who are working hard to regain continence. However, by managing fluid intake to accommodate your schedule, the extra bathroom trips will not be an inconvenience.

Drink extra fluid during those parts of the day when you have easy access to a bathroom. In the work environment, this may mean drinking water or some other beverage shortly before your lunch break. Another trick is to refrain from drinking until you return from shopping or from some other activity that puts a big distance between you and the bathroom.

Limiting your extra fluid intake to daytime hours should prevent having to make frequent nighttime trips to the toilet. Many women find that restricting liquids after eating dinner works well for them. It is commonly observed that drinking caffeine-free beverages with your evening meal and avoiding artificial sweeteners are other helpful tactics.

Having *diabetes* can also affect urination patterns. When you have high blood sugar, you need to urinate more often because there is more water in your urine. Carefully monitoring your diet, blood sugar, and diabetes medication can greatly improve this situation. Producing large amounts of nearly colorless urine may indicate that your blood sugar is too high.

Some women take water pills, or *diuretics*, to help control *high blood pressure* and the water weight gain, and edema (swelling) caused by heart disease. Taking diuretics containing furosemide (Lasix), triamterene (Dyrenium), and hydrochlorothiazide (this has multiple brand names but is best known as HCTZ) will also make you lose more water. However, to protect your cardiovascular health, it is important to follow your doctor's instructions and take prescribed diuretics.

Scheduling the timing of your water pills can make a big difference. Taking them in the morning or in the afternoon as a way to reschedule your bedtime dose can prevent you from making nighttime trips to the toilet. Some women who take diuretics tend to accumulate water in their legs and feet. Putting your feet up for a few hours late in the day helps you eliminate fluids before you go to bed. This works by redistributing the excess fluid that has gathered in your feet and legs back into your bloodstream. The fluid is then filtered through your kidneys and deposited in your bladder so you can eliminate it before you go to bed—rather than in the middle of the night! Medications, such as *antihistamines* to treat allergies and *sedatives* and *tranquilizers* used to treat anxiety, may also cause people to produce more urine. Just like timing your diuretics to minimize urinary inconvenience, you can schedule these medications conveniently as well. Be sure to check with your doctor before altering when you take your medicines.

Foods and Beverages that Can Make Bladder Control More Difficult

Eating certain foods can make bladder control more difficult for some women. Caffeine and *oxalate*, both compounds plants make, are examples of two naturally occurring substances associated with increased overactive bladder symptoms. Caffeine is thought to be both a stimulant and a bladder irritant and perhaps even a mild diuretic. Consuming caffeinated beverages can worsen mild incontinence and make it more difficult to manage. In addition to coffee and tea, foods such as chocolate and cocoa also contain caffeine and caffeinelike compounds.

Although women vary in their bladder sensitivities, many find that eliminating foods that naturally contain large amounts of oxalate reduces urge and improves bladder control (see table 4.2). A surprising number of foods, ranging from peanuts to tofu and strawberries, contain oxalate. In addition to causing irritable bladder symptoms, oxalate is also associated with the formation of urinary tract stones throughout the urinary tract and *urogenital* tract pain.

Some women discover associations between other foods and increases in bladder irritation symptoms. Because not everybody responds in the same way, you will need to discover which foods and beverages you need to avoid. Foods and beverages commonly associated with bladder irritation, for varied reasons, include the following:

- Carbonated beverages, including sparkling water
- Alcoholic beverages
- Milk and other dairy products
- Coffee and tea—even if decaffeinated
- Citrus juices such as orange juice and grapefruit juice
- Tomatoes and other tomato-based products such as spaghetti sauce
- Highly spiced foods such as those that contain chili pepper or curry
- Sugar, honey, corn syrup, and artificial sweeteners

This may seem like a long list, but eliminating several of these foods, spices, or beverages might make your symptoms much more manageable.

Table 4.2. Avoiding High-Oxalate Foods
Can Reduce Urge Incontinence

Examples of High-Oxalate Foods	Examples of Low-Oxalate Foods
Draft beer	Bottled beer
Tea	Buttermilk
Cocoa	Milk
Peanuts and peanut butter	Yogurt with low oxalate fruits
Tofu	Eggs
Beans	Cheeses
Beets	Beef, lamb, and pork
Celery	Chicken
Chives	Fish and shellfish
Collards	Avocados
Eggplant	Brussels sprouts
Leeks	Cauliflower
Okra	Cabbage
Sweet potatoes	Mushrooms
Spinach	Onions
Lemon, lime and orange peels and juices	Green peas
Rhubarb	White potatoes
Strawberries	Radishes
Tangerines	Apples
Wheat germ	Bananas
Almonds	Bing cherries
Cashews	Melons
Walnuts	Nectarines
Tomatoes and foods that contain tomatoes	Peaches
	Plums
	Cereals
	Noodles
	Rice
	Bread
	Vegetable oils, butter, and margarine
	Jams and jellies made with low-oxalate fruits

Dietary Fiber

There are many reasons why consuming dietary fiber is a health-promoting habit. Eating enough dietary fiber helps make soft stools that easily pass through the intestines. This reduces excessive pressure on the pelvic floor muscles when having a bowel movement can improve continence by maintaining pelvic floor muscle strength.

Scientists have also discovered that eating a fiber-rich diet improves heart health by removing artery-clogging cholesterol from our bodies. Eating dietary fiber may also be an important factor in reducing colon cancer risk.

A diet rich in fiber-containing foods is a good weight-loss strategy. Because we cannot digest fiber, it is not a source of calories. Eating fiber-rich foods, as long as they are not fried or smothered in sauces or salad dressing, allows us to feel full and satisfied without a high caloric intake.

There are two types of dietary fiber. Insoluble fiber does not dissolve in water. Insoluble fiber includes cellulose, the substance in plant cell walls and the woody materials that make plants resistant to breaking. Foods that are good sources of insoluble fiber include fresh fruits and vegetables and whole grains such as wheat, rye, and wheat bran (fig. 4.2).

Soluble fiber combines with water. When cooked, foods that contain soluble fiber make a gummy substance. Some good sources of soluble fiber include oats, beans, and barley. If you have noticed a gluey material in a pot of boiled oatmeal or in the liquid that accompanies canned beans, then you know exactly what soluble fiber looks like!

Nutrition researchers recommend that people consume twenty to thirty-five grams or about one ounce of dietary fiber each day. The fact that most people in the United States get only ten to fifteen grams in their daily diet indicates our dependence on processed and overrefined foods.

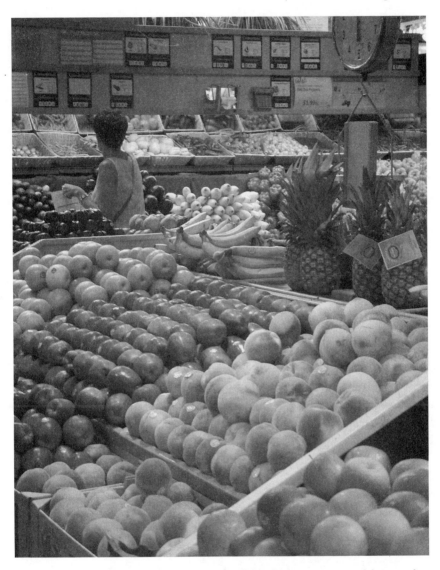

Fig. 4.2. A variety of fresh fruits, vegetables, and whole grains in your diet is a good way to increase your daily fiber consumption.

Rather than eating more grains, fresh fruits, and vegetables, many people opt to using fiber supplements to manage constipation problems. However, many high-fiber foods such as beans and peas actually contain more fiber per serving than a single fiber supplement portion. This means that people need to consume large amounts of fiber supplements to get sufficiently soft and bulky stools. Most clinicians recommend getting dietary bulk from real food sources.

It is important to introduce high-fiber foods gradually into your diet over a period of three to four weeks. Suddenly eating large amounts of dietary fiber can lead to intestinal discomfort, bloating, and gas. It is also important to eat foods that will supply both types of fiber. Here are some simple ways to increase both kinds of fiber in your diet:

- Eat fresh fruits rather than drinking fruit juices
- Eat fresh vegetables
- Replace some servings of white bread and processed cereal with breads and cereals that contain bran or whole grains

By now you realize that like most Americans, you are probably not getting enough bulky fiber in your daily diet. However, you are probably also wondering what you actually need to do to make sure that you are consuming at least twenty grams of fiber on a daily basis.

The Dietary Guidelines for Americans suggests that each day we eat:

- Three or more servings of vegetables
- Two or more servings of fresh fruit
- Six or more servings of grain products

Use the information in table 4.4 to convert servings to actual quantities. Maximize your daily fiber by frequently choosing whole-

Table 4.3. Some High-Fiber Foods and Ways to Use Them

High-Fiber Food	Ways to Use Them
Black beans, kidney beans, split peas, lentils, garbanzo beans, pinto beans	Soups, salads, spreads
Bran cereals	Breakfast cereal, muffins
Fresh or frozen lima beans	Vegetable serving, soups
Fresh or frozen green peas	Vegetable serving, salads, soups
Dried figs, apricots, and dates	Dessert or a snack, add to baked goods, oatmeal topping
Raspberries, blackberries, and strawberries	Fruit serving, fruit salad, fruit smoothie, sorbet or ice cream serving
Sweet corn, fresh, canned, or frozen	Vegetable serving, salads, soups
Whole wheat and other whole grains such as rye, oats, cornmeal	Breads, muffins, pancakes, pasta, pizza crust
Broccoli	Vegetable serving, salad, soup, baked potato topping
Baked or boiled potatoes with skin	Baked, soup, salad

grain breads and pasta. Replacing white rice with brown rice is another helpful strategy.

Before changing your diet, it is a good idea to self-assess your current eating habits. Use Worksheet 4D and the information contained in tables 4.3 and 4.4 to evaluate the specific dietary changes that will efficiently increase your daily fiber intake. Read food labels or use the Internet and search phrases and words such as "dietary fiber," and the specific food name and "fiber" to discover the fiber content of foods not included in table 4.3. Before long, making fiber-rich food choices will come naturally to you.

Table 4.4. Servings to Quantity Conversions

Type of Food	Number of Servings per Day	Amount of Food for a Single Serving
Vegetables	3 or more	Leafy green vegetables: 1 cup Other vegetables: ½ cup Cooked beans or peas: ½ cup
Fruits	2 or more	1 Medium apple, orange, or banana Canned fruit: ½ cup
Grain products such as bread, pasta, cereal, rice	6 or more	Bread: 1 slice Bun, bagel, English muffin –½ Dry cereal: ¾ cup Cooked cereal: ½ cup Rice or pasta: ½ cup

HEALTHY WEIGHT

Being too heavy is a stress incontinence risk factor because excess weight increases pressure on your pelvic floor muscles. You do not have to lose large amounts of weight to make stress incontinence more manageable. Research shows that losing as few as ten pounds can make bladder control easier for you. Maintaining a healthy weight can also reduce your risk for other health problems that include heart disease, diabetes, and wear and tear on the knees and feet.

Cutting down on food portion size is a good way to begin your weight-loss program. Eating a variety of foods in moderation is also helpful. By doing this, you will develop lifelong healthy eating habits.

Exercise is another helpful weight-control strategy. Walking, bicycling, and swimming are examples of low-impact activities that people of all ages can enjoy. Some women avoid exercise because it makes them leak urine more. Using absorbency products or a pessary while exercising can help break this negative cycle. Keeping physically active also reduces constipation problems and improves the overall sense of wellness.

SMOKING

Smoking is another important incontinence risk factor. Research shows an association between stress and urge incontinence and cigarette smoking. In fact, women smokers are nearly 30 percent more likely to have incontinence problems than women who do not smoke. Researchers believe that cigarette smoke contains substances that are bladder irritants and contribute to urge incontinence. Other cigarette smoke substances may damage muscle tissue and worsen stress incontinence.

Smoker's cough also aggravates stress incontinence when coughing puts excess pressure on pelvic floor muscles. When smokers quit smoking, they often see improvement in their ability to manage urge and stress incontinence symptoms.

In addition to incontinence, smoking is a risk factor for heart disease and cervical cancer, and it worsens certain diabetic problems. Cigarette smoke compounds can also make your *immune system* less able to fight disease.

MAINTAINING AN ACTIVE LIFESTYLE

Clinical research confirms what you already know. Having incontinence problems is frustrating, embarrassing, and compromises your quality of life. Many women, even those who have small urine leaks, find it difficult to enjoy sex with their partner, socialize, or leave the house for work or shopping. Social and emotional isolation can lead to depression and a self-perception of poor health.

While the "first step" methods described in this chapter may reduce or even eliminate urine leaks, finding what works takes time and patience. Until you discover the combinations of pelvic floor exercises, scheduled urination, and dietary changes that work best for you, absorbency products and careful wardrobe planning can reduce embarrassing events. This can help you feel more comfortable working with your colleagues and socializing with friends and family members.

Absorbency Products

Absorbency products, just like the tampons and pads used to absorb menstrual blood, allow women to maintain a comfortably active lifestyle. Using absorbent pads, panty liners, disposable briefs, and reusable incontinence products give you the confidence and freedom to leave the house. Steve, an incontinence product distributor, reinforces this idea by saying, "Briefs are becoming more absorbent and less crinkly because today's incontinent baby boomer still wants to play tennis." They are also an important factor in helping you stick with your pelvic floor exercise and scheduled urination programs.

Many women resist using absorbency products because they are afraid that wearing them will draw attention to their incontinence problem. They believe people will notice clothing that fits differently. Maybe others will even hear something that draws their attention. However, as one disposable brief user aptly states, "People look at smiles not at bottoms."

Because urinary incontinence is so common, you will not be the first among your friends and family to use urinary incontinence products. There are many types of absorbency products for you to choose from. While many women use sanitary napkins and minipads to manage urine leaks, they are not always the best choice. These products, designed to absorb blood, do not satisfactorily retain large amounts of urine.

Sanitary napkins and minipads do not keep urine away from your skin. Using them without frequent changes may cause painful skin irritation, open sores, and infections. Sanitary napkins and pads also do not control urine odors.

Disposable incontinence products are specifically designed to absorb and retain urine. Urinary incontinence products contain wood pulp and a polymer. The wood pulp increases absorbency and the polymer, by converting liquid urine into a gel, minimizes the leaks and odors.

Although sanitary napkins and minipads are comparatively less expensive, they do not work as well as urine-absorbency products. For women who experience urinary dampness or who leak only while participating in certain activities, using these products can be helpful. When wetness and skin irritations necessitate frequent pad changes, reusable (cloth) absorbency products may actually be the more economical choice.

Once you make the decision to give urinary incontinence supplies a try, you will discover there are many products to choose from. Similar to purchases of tampons and sanitary pads, women buy specific absorbency products to accommodate for "high- and low-flow" situations. There are also many styles—allowing you to buy the best protection for your body weight, activity level, and travel needs. By trying different products you will find styles that also fit comfortably and inconspicuously under your clothing (table 4.5 Disposable Pad Tips; figs. 4.3a, b, c).

Some women prefer using reusable pads and undergarments. Item for item, they are more expensive than disposable absorbency products, but they are often less expensive over the long term. Most manufacturers guarantee reusable pads and undergarments to last between one hundred to two hundred washings. In addition to potential cost benefits, reusable absorbency products have a more natural fit, are less bulky to store, and do not create disposal problems. Many women who use reusable pads and garments opt for disposable ones when spending extended time away from home or when traveling. Doing this means they do not have to worry about storing and washing reusable pads (table 4.6).

Although you can buy absorbency products at just about any store that carries healthcare goods, the Internet is another excellent resource. Using keyword phrases such as "incontinence products," "urinary incontinence products," "absorbency products," and "adult disposable underwear" is an efficient and discreet way to learn about incontinence aids in the privacy of your own home.

Many Web sites have chat rooms where women can get helpful

Fig. 4.3. By trying different absorbency products you will find the styles that prevent leaks and fit comfortably and inconspicuously under your clothing.

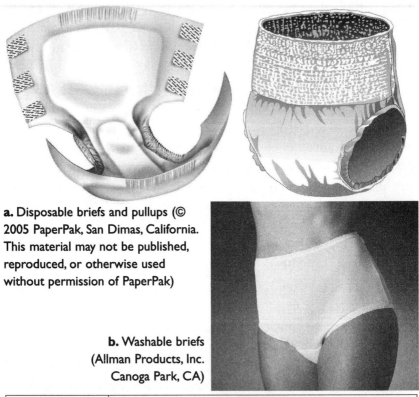

a. Disposable briefs and pullups (© 2005 PaperPak, San Dimas, California. This material may not be published, reproduced, or otherwise used without permission of PaperPak)

b. Washable briefs (Allman Products, Inc. Canoga Park, CA)

FIND USER'S HEIGHT & WEIGHT:										WEIGHT IN POUNDS																								
HEIGHT	85	90	95	100	105	110	115	120	125	130	135	140	145	150	155	160	165	170	175	180	185	190	195	200	205	210	215	220	225	230	235	240	245	250
4' 10"																																		
4' 11"																																		
5' 0"																																		
5' 1"																																		
5' 2"																																		
5' 3"																																		
5' 4"																																		
5' 5"																																		
5' 6"																																		
5' 7"																																		
5' 8"																																		
5' 9"																																		
5' 10"																																		
5' 11"																																		
6' 0"																																		
6' 1"																																		
6' 2"																																		

c. Using a sizing chart such as this one will help you find the absorbency briefs that fit well and are less likely to leak (© 2005 PaperPak, San Dimas, California. This material may not be published, reproduced, or otherwise used without permission of PaperPak)

Table 4.5. Disposable Pads: Helpful Tips

- Buy a small quantity until you are sure the product works for you
- Manufacturer absorbency claims are not always comparable
- You can wear two or more pads for extra protection, but only the outer one should have a waterproof backing
- Snug fitting pants help keep pads in position
- Smaller pads with an adhesive strip are easier to keep in place, but are only suitable for small urine losses
- Carry a plastic grocery store bag so that you can easily dispose of used pads

---

hints from experienced product users. Some Internet stores offer trial packages that include a variety of absorbency products. If you decide to order absorbency products online, many companies promise they will arrive at your home in an unmarked box.

Skin Care

Although keeping the urogenital area dry and clean is important, you need to also take special care to prevent skin breakdown and infections. Vigorous washing and using harsh soaps can make the skin sore, rough, and dry. This increases your chances of getting an infection.

Using incontinence skin cleansers that are pH-balanced, no-rinse, fragrance-free, alcohol-free, and residue-free can help prevent this painful outcome. It is also important to avoid wearing excessively tight undergarments and clothing. Although some women wear tight garments to prevent leaks, tight clothing can create the warm and wet conditions that increase bacterial growth and the risk of infection.

You can find out more about incontinence skin cleansers from your local pharmacist, hospital supply salesperson, or from the Internet. The phrase "incontinence skin cleansers" is a good way to begin your Internet research. Similar to absorbency products, you can purchase these skincare products online.

Table 4.6. Reusable Pads and Undergarments: Helpful Tips

- Reusable pads and undergarments may be more expensive to buy, but less expensive than disposable products in the long-run
- Usually guaranteed to last for 100 to 200 washings
- Wash a few times before using to soften fabric and improve absorbency
- Rinse used pads and undergarments as soon as possible
- Store rinsed washable pads and undergarments in an airtight bucket of cold water before washing
- Avoid using bleach and fabric softeners because they can damage fabric and reduce absorbency
- Do not overload your washer
- Follow manufacturers' instructions concerning type of detergent and washing and drying temperatures
- After drying make sure that both the "stay dry" surface and the absorbant core are dry
- Air before putting cleaned pads and undergarments away
- Store with absorbent layer facing outwards

Controlling Odor

Normal urine is mostly water and urea—a substance our body makes in the process of digesting the proteins we eat. Fresh urine normally does not have an offensive odor. Some people describe the odor of fresh urine as "salty like the ocean."

Once exposed to air and the bacteria living in the urogenital area, urine does become smelly. The combination of oxygen and bacterial activity converts urea into ammonia. This substance has a strong and offensive smell and also irritates the skin.

Managing your fluid intake can help reduce odor problems. Concentrated urine has a stronger and therefore more noticeable salty odor than urine that contains enough water. Drinking water can also help lower your risk for getting bladder infections.

When you do have a bladder infection, not only does this worsen urgency, it also gives the *bacteria* living in your bladder the opportunity to make the urine often smelly even before you excrete it. With a bladder infection, urine smells "musty."

Eating certain foods can produce strong-smelling urine. The classic odor-producing food is asparagus. In about 50 percent of people, eating asparagus causes them to make urine that some describe as smelling "woodsy" or perhaps even a little "skunky."

In addition to bathing, it is also necessary to frequently replace wet absorbency pads and undergarments with fresh ones. Some absorbency products contain odor-reducing substances. Wiping the urogenital area with adult wipes—not baby wipes—is another way to control odor. Unlike baby wipes, adult wipes are larger and contain odor-reducing and skincare ingredients. Using them both reduces odor and skin irritation problems (fig. 4.4).

Washing clothing, sheets, and reusable absorbency products is another concern. Once urine dries, its odor tends to linger—even after washing. Many women recommend rinsing wet clothing and cloth absorbency products and storing them in a bucket with a lid until you are ready to wash them, as is done with cloth diapers for babies.

Using a detergent that contains enzymes that remove blood and other body fluids is helpful. Hospital supply personnel recommend adding enzyme-based products, normally used to remove pet stains and odors from rugs, to your laundry load. You can buy these products in pet and animal supply stores.

Clothing Strategies

Making good clothing choices can help hide and prevent accidents. Peggy, an incontinence nurse specialist, often remarks at how nicely dressed her patients are. Even though many of them have little or no bladder control, they have found ways to dress that do not draw attention to wet spots or to bulky undergarments. Based on what her patients tell her, Peggy suggests wearing darker clothes—navy blue,

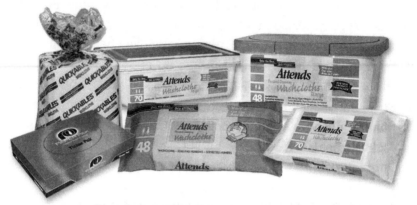

Fig. 4.4. Adult wipes contain odor-reducing and skincare ingredients. (© 2005 PaperPak, San Dimas, California. This material may not be published, reproduced, or otherwise used without permission of PaperPak)

dark brown, and black—as a good way to disguise wet marks. You can discover which colors and fabric types work best by wetting them with a water-soaked sponge or washcloth. Wearing long shirts, sweaters, and tunic tops is another way to camouflage wet spots and some of the bulkier types of undergarments.

It is also important to consider how quickly you can undress. Avoid wearing pantyhose, tights, and clothing with difficult buttons, clasps, or zippers. You do not want a tricky button or belt buckle to foil your scheduled urination exercise program!

Traveling Strategies

With a little preparation you can easily travel to work, the store, or even take a trip to the Grand Canyon. Many incontinence patients say they carry a comfortable backpack or sling bag packed with absorbency supplies, cleanup products, and sometimes a change of clothing. They also say it is important to bring plastic bags, like the ones used to pack groceries, so you can easily and discreetly dispose of wet pads and other absorbency products or to transport wet clothing home. Resealable plastic bags are a good way to transport a supply of adult wipes. One woman reports that she likes to bring some newspaper with her. This way, if she needs to change her clothes she does not have to stand directly on the restroom floor. To make your travel bag manageable, store extra absorbency products and clothing in the car.

And What about Sex?

Urine leaks while having sex is a common problem for women who have stress and urge incontinence. However, there are many things you can do that will reduce the chances of losing urine during intercourse. Taking medication to reduce overactive bladder symptoms may make urge symptoms less of a problem. Emptying your bladder before sex is a helpful practice for women who have urge and stress incontinence. Using a vaginal lubricant and positioning yourself either under or alongside your partner lessens physical stress on your bladder and pelvic floor. And since keeping your bed dry during intercourse is another common concern, use an absorbent bed pad to protect your sheets and mattress. Be sure to remember these "PEARLs" so that urinary incontinence does not sexually isolate you from your partner:

- Position yourself on your back or side
- Empty your bladder
- Absorbent pads to protect your sheets and mattress
- Rx—use your prescriptions to reduce overactive bladder symptoms
- Lubricants are another way to reduce physical stress on your bladder and pelvic floor

NOW WHAT HAPPENS?

For many of you, these "first step" techniques will improve continence to the extent that incontinence no longer affects your lifestyle. Others will discover that you have less urgency, wetness, and fewer incidents where leaking is a problem. To help prolong or even maintain this level of continence it is important that you continue doing pelvic floor exercises and make these newly acquired diet and fluid management strategies lifelong habits. And if overactive bladder and urgency returns, you may have to "remind" your bladder about good behavior with another scheduled urination exercise session!

Unfortunately, these "first steps" do not help all women to the extent they desire or need to manage an active lifestyle. If this is your situation, consider seeking medical help.

A significant number of women do not have easy access to medical care. Lack of insurance coverage is a problem for others and living far away from a comprehensive medical facility can make finding specialized care difficult. Even if you face these challenges, medical care is available in regional medical centers and clinics linked to medical research and teaching institutions.

In the next chapter, you will learn how to find the best medical care and how to communicate with your doctor and the other health professionals you may see. We will also show you how to find and take advantage of continence support groups and other information resources.

WORKSHEETS

Worksheet 4A: Voiding Diary

This chart is a record of your fluid intake, voiding, and urine leakage. Choose any three days (entire twenty-four-hour periods) to complete this record. They do not have to be three days in a row. Choose days when you can measure *every* void. Using the example given on the following page, begin recording upon rising in the morning. A review of your voiding diary will help you understand your urination habits. Showing this information to your doctor will make it easier for the both of you to talk about urinary incontinence.

Day 1

Time	Amount Voided (use a spare measuring cup or a plastic urine collection "hat" available at medical supply stores)	Leak Volume 0=dry 1=drops/damp 2=wet soaked 3=bladder emptied	Activity During Leak	Was There Urge?	Fluid Intake
7:00 AM	1/2 cup	2	Running	Yes	
8:15 AM					1 cup herbal tea
8:45 AM		3	Standing up	No	

Day 2

Time	Amount Voided (use a spare measuring cup or a plastic urine collection "hat" available at medical supply stores)	Leak Volume 0=dry 1=drops/damp 2=wet soaked 3=bladder emptied	Activity During Leak	Was There Urge?	Fluid Intake

Day 3

Time	Amount Voided (use a spare measuring cup or a plastic urine collection "hat" available at medical supply stores)	Leak Volume 0=dry 1=drops/damp 2=wet soaked 3=bladder emptied	Activity During Leak	Was There Urge?	Fluid Intake

Worksheet 4B: Pelvic Floor Exercise Diary

Using the example given below, record the position, type, and number of pelvic floor exercises you do each day. Doing pelvic floor exercises on a daily basis helps strengthen your pelvic floor muscles and reduces urine leaks caused by stress incontinence. If urgency is a problem, remember a couple of quick flicks can provide relief.

Date	Time	Position	Quick Flick Sets*	Squeeze†
June 28	7:30 AM	Sitting	12	4
June 29	4:30 PM	Standing	10	3

*One "quick flick"—is squeeze, hold, and relax
†Squeeze—the time contracted in seconds

Worksheet 4C: Scheduled Urination Exercises

Make a chart similar to the one below to help you organize your scheduled urination exercises. If necessary, you can begin using shorter time intervals than one hour. Remember, your voiding schedule begins when you awake in the morning and continues until you go to bed at night. You may increase the time between voidings as your bladder adjusts to holding urine for longer periods.

Time:	Feel urge?	What you did to control urge:	Did it work?
7:00 AM	Yes	PFE*	Yes
8:00 AM	No		
9:00 AM	Yes	Sat down	No
		PFE	Yes

*Pelvic Floor Exercise

Worksheet 4D: Evaluating Your Diet for Fiber Content

Consuming twenty to thirty-five grams of fiber each day improves health in many ways. Getting a sense of how much fiber you eat each day will help you make the dietary changes needed to reach this goal.

The Top High-Fiber Foods*

Food	Portion	Grams fiber
Dried beans, peas, and other legumes	Cooked kidney beans: I cup	16
	Cooked split peas: I cup	16
	Cooked pinto beans: I cup	14
	Cooked black beans: I cup	15
Bran cereals	Bran Buds: 1/2 cup	10.4
	Raisin Bran: I cup	7.2
	Instant oatmeal: I cup	3.9
	Old-fashioned oatmeal: I cup	8
Fresh or frozen lima beans	1/2 cup	5.8
Fresh or frozen green peas	1/2 cup	8.8
Dried fruit	Figs: 2	3.7
	Dates: 2	1.7
	Apricots: 2 halves	1.7
	Raisins: I cup	5.4
	Prunes: 3	1.9
	Dates: I cup	14.2
Berries	Raspberries: I cup	11
	Strawberries: I cup	3.3
	Blackberries: 1/2 cup	4.4
Sweet corn	I medium ear	2.2
Whole-grain foods	2 slices whole-grain bread	6
	I cup whole-grain flours such as rye, cornmeal, and buckwheat	12-14
Cooked soy beans	I cup	10.3
Baked potato with skin	Small baked potato	4.6
	Sweet potato	4.8
Frozen mixed vegetables	I cup	8
Fresh plums, pears, and apples with skin	I	3.3
Greens	Spinach: I cup	7
	Beet greens, kale, collards: 1/2 cup	4
Nuts	Almonds, peanuts, and walnuts: 1/4 cup	2.4
Fresh cherries	10	1.2
Banana	I medium	3
Raw carrots	1/4 cup	1.7
Cooked carrots	1/2 cup	3.4
Coconut meat	I tablespoon	1.7
Brussels sprouts	3/4 cup	3

*It is interesting to note that a single serving of most dietary fiber supplements (I tablespoon) contains only 3.4 grams of fiber. A single medium-sized carrot also contains this amount.

Day 1	Foods Eaten	Amounts	Grams Fiber
Breakfast			
Lunch			
Dinner			
Snacks			
Day 2			
Breakfast			
Lunch			
Dinner			
Snacks			
Day 3			
Breakfast			
Lunch			
Dinner			
Snacks			
Day 4			
Breakfast			
Lunch			
Dinner			
Snacks			
Day 5			
Breakfast			
Lunch			
Dinner			
Snacks			
Day 6			
Breakfast			
Lunch			
Dinner			
Snacks			
Day 7			
Breakfast			
Lunch			
Dinner			
Snacks			

FREQUENTLY ASKED QUESTIONS

1. Do I have to do pelvic floor exercises forever?

Yes, doing pelvic floor exercises on a daily basis will help you maintain your improvement in pelvic floor strength. In fact, many doctors recommend that all women do daily pelvic floor exercises, whether they have urinary continence problems or not.

2. Do I have to do scheduled urination exercises forever?

No. However, if you notice a return or an increase in urge incontinence symptoms, doing another session of scheduled urination exercises will help you reestablish good brain-bladder communication.

3. Do I really have to drink six to eight glasses of water every day?

You should consume the equivalent of six to eight glasses of water every day to maintain good hydration and to reduce constipation. Remember that this volume, equaling 1.5 to 2 quarts of fluid, also includes the milk you consume with your breakfast cereal; the moisture contained in fruits, vegetables, and other foods; and all the beverages you consume during the day.

4. There seem to be so many foods that cause bladder irritability. How do I decide which ones I really need to avoid?

It is a long list! Fortunately, most women will discover that out of all of these foods, only a few cause problems for them. Look at the list and then think about which foods you frequently eat. Can you associate any of these with increases in bladder urge sensations? Go through the list again and find the foods you occasionally eat. Can you associate any of them with increases in bladder urge sensations?

If you believe spaghetti sauce, chili peppers, coffee, orange juice, and cola drinks cause problems, then avoid all of them for a few days and see if you are doing better. To discover which ones are the real culprits, over the course of several days add one at a time back into your diet. Doing this might reveal that orange juice is the only food you need to avoid.

5. I am a diabetic. How do I increase dietary fiber without also making my blood sugar too high?

Clinical research shows that a very high fiber diet (50 grams) plays an important role in helping type-2 (non-insulin dependent) diabetics control their blood sugar. However, you should talk to your doctor before making dietary changes that have the potential to affect your blood sugar or your diabetes medications.

6. How long will it take for treatments to work?

This will depend on many factors, including how long you have had bladder control problems, the cause and severity of your condition, and how thoroughly you are able to incorporate these first steps into daily life. Like any other lifestyle or health adjustment you might make, bladder control treatment results happen at different rates for everyone. We are pleased to tell you that the vast majority of women who begin treatment for urinary incontinence see an improvement in their symptoms within a few weeks to several months. While this may seem like a long time to wait for results, it is a short time compared to the many years some women have endured bladder leakage.

7. What can I do if none of these "first step" methods improve my urge or stress incontinence problems?

If pelvic floor and scheduled urination exercises and changes in dietary and smoking habits do not help, you need to talk to your healthcare provider. However, consider showing your clinician your completed worksheets. This information will show them what you have tried and your results. It will also help them make good "next step" decisions.

CHAPTER 5

GETTING THE HELP YOU WANT

"I didn't need to worry about this.
My doctor listened and was helpful."
Dee—recalling her first visit with a doctor
about bladder control

OFF TO A GOOD START

Theresa, newly retired, had decided it was time to see a doctor about her troublesome overactive bladder symptoms. Although retirement now gave her the time to enjoy fishing trips with her husband, she knew her sudden uncontrollable bladder urges would make their trips impossible.

Having recently moved, she was concerned about discussing something so private with a new doctor. After asking her friends for their suggestions, she made an appointment with a nearby primary care physician that they recommended. Although she had hoped to find a woman doctor, she was glad that she was finally able to find a doctor willing to take new patients. "I just hope this doctor will take the time to answer my questions and I hope I can understand the answers," she told her husband. Her biggest question was how soon she could get relief.

Before her first appointment, Theresa realized that she felt a little nervous. As she described her symptoms during the appointment she worried that she might forget some important detail. She felt better when the doctor repeated her statements to make sure he understood her symptoms.

Theresa's doctor first did a simple urine test to make sure a bladder infection wasn't causing or contributing to her urgency. Because the results of that test showed she didn't have an infection, Theresa's doctor gave her a prescription for a medication to help reduce bladder urgency. He also talked with her about how to do pelvic floor exercises to help offset her overwhelming urges. He explained that these approaches were only the beginning of her treatment and referred her to a urogynecologist for further evaluation of her condition. Although Theresa's primary care doctor had been a good listener, it was a brief visit. While the doctor couldn't say exactly how long it would take Theresa to get better, she was pleased she had already made some progress. She hoped the urogynecologist would be as easy to talk with and understand. After making an appointment, she told her husband, "I think we're getting closer to a fishing trip!"

STARTING THE CONVERSATION

Talking with a doctor about bladder control problems is one of the most important things you can do to improve continence. In doing so, you open the door to understanding your treatment options. Unfortunately, many women do not believe telling their doctor about their bladder control difficulties will be helpful. Many others do not feel comfortable bringing up this embarrassing topic. Still others just never "get around to it."

Even with a doctor you know quite well, talking about bladder control difficulties can feel awkward. Do not wait for your doctor to bring up the issue of poor bladder control. In many cases, doctors do not ask their female patients about it. Either they do not know to ask, or they believe a woman would mention the topic herself.

In this chapter you will learn about getting the bladder control help you want through effective communication with the doctors and other healthcare providers you will meet during your urinary incontinence treatment process. You will also learn about using resources such as support groups and the Internet as ways of getting help.

FINDING A DOCTOR, GETTING A REFERRAL

Often women see their *nurse practitioner*, family doctor, primary care provider, gynecologist, or they visit a community health clinic when they first decide to seek treatment. Women may choose to bring up bladder control issues during a visit to their family doctor regarding other health issues or during a routine checkup. Depending on your symptoms and local health facility options the primary care doctor may refer you to a specialist, a physical therapist, or a surgeon who specializes in urinary incontinence surgery. Women who do not have a primary care doctor or a gynecologist can find help at a local community health center, county hospital, or nearby university teaching hospital.

YOUR FIRST VISIT

Because many types of healthcare providers treat urinary incontinence and pelvic floor disorders, your "first visit" for bladder control problems may actually be one of several first visits. For each of these appointments bring your list of questions, talk to the nurse about your condition, and be prepared to talk openly with the doctor or other medical professional. By showing an active interest in your care, you will lay a foundation for productive communication.

An appointment for bladder control problems will begin much like any other doctor appointment. You will be asked to fill out a medical history form in the waiting area. Then the nurse will escort you to the exam room, take your blood pressure, weight, height, temperature, pulse, and ask why you are visiting the doctor. When the doctor arrives, he or she will ask questions about your medical history. In addition to a list of symptoms and questions, be sure to bring a list of your medications, other medical conditions, and surgeries you have had. This way, you can quickly and thoroughly provide the background information your nurse and doctor need.

As your doctor asks about your symptoms, provide detailed, candid answers. Be sure to tell your doctor about any symptoms such as frequent day and night time trips to the bathroom that you are having that he or she does not bring up. Do not assume a symptom is unimportant because the doctor does not ask about it.

After the first appointment, depending on what is found, the doctor may suggest certain medical tests to help diagnose your condition or recommend certain treatments. Your doctor may also refer you to another healthcare provider such as a gynecologist, a urogynecologist, a urologist, or a physical therapist for further diagnostic testing and/or treatment.

HELPING YOUR DOCTOR HELP YOU

From the beginning, your doctor is counting on you to provide the information needed to make a diagnosis and plan treatment. Tell your doctor about your experiences with any of the first-step approaches you have tried from chapter 4. Bring along any worksheets from chapters 2 and 4 that you have completed. The improvement, or lack of improvement, in symptoms will give your

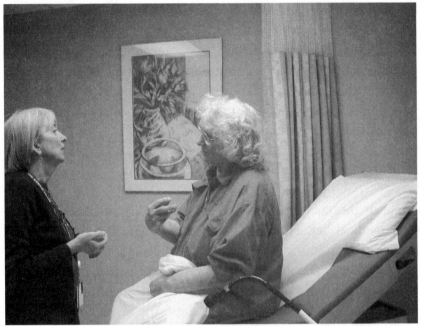

Fig. 5.1. Talking openly with your doctor or other healthcare professional is an important part of your treatment process.

doctor important clues about your condition. It may also help the doctor more efficiently plan a treatment approach for you (fig. 5.1).

Sometimes, without realizing it, patients make it more difficult for their doctor to understand their health issues and provide the best care for them. In fact, a common problem doctors face is that some patients "clam up" during the appointment. These patients feel that the physician is in charge of the appointment and should do all the talking. This is simply not the case. If you begin to feel like a "passenger" rather than a "driver" in your treatment plan, do what you can to participate more in this important conversation. Remember, it's *your body*. You have the bladder leakage problem. You want to control it. If you don't say something, the doctor may not be able to give you the help you need and want.

Another common problem is that some patients believe it's the doctor's job to know or guess what is wrong based on a few simple statements. Behaviors such as "clamming up" and "withholding information" are unfair and interfere with the doctor's ability to treat you effectively! You will get the best treatment if you team up with your doctor, participate in your appointments, and remember that healthcare providers are not mind readers.

Understanding Your Treatment Process

Some of the many factors that affect bladder treatments include your medical history, age, as well as type and severity of symptoms. Other factors include your physician's training and the medical facilities available to you. Because every patient and her treatment situation are unique, think of your treatment process as a "custom job"! Just because your best friend had surgery that improved her continence does not mean the same combination of treatments will work for you. Even if you both have bladder control symptoms that appear the same, do not expect the same treatment plans. If you know someone who is happy with her treatment, you can ask your doctor if it is a good option for you. Do not be surprised if the answer is no or "I don't know that answer yet."

Something else to keep in mind is the difference between improving continence and curing incontinence. Your doctor and the other specialists you see offer treatments that may improve or eliminate nearly all of your symptoms. However, "cure" is not a word that applies to all urinary incontinence treatments. Bladder control problems result from changes in the anatomy and function of your urinary and pelvic organs and tissues. Your doctor and other healthcare providers can only improve—not replace—how your bladder and other related organs and tissues work and function together.

When you begin to seek treatment for poor bladder control, you will probably want to know how long it will take. Ask general questions about the treatment process and the outlook for improvement, but do not expect your doctor to predict specific details. Remember, while patients may respond somewhat differently to treatment, you can, however, expect improvement. The good news is that most women do get better with bladder control treatment. How long it might take and the amount of improvement is not always easily determined.

WHAT DOES "BETTER BLADDER CONTROL" MEAN TO YOU?

Come to your appointment ready to talk about what "better bladder control" really means to you. Even if your doctor doesn't ask you directly, be sure to mention treatment goals such as reducing urgency so that you can concentrate better at work or travel without having to worry about bladder accidents.

You might wonder why talking about treatment goals is important. After all—isn't reestablishing the bladder function you remember having earlier in life the only goal? Unfortunately, this is not realistic. When doctors talk about successful incontinence treatments, they really mean one of two things—making it easier for you to manage incontinence or doing something that makes leaking less likely.

Describing your goals and using personal milestones as reference points are often effective communication tactics. Some women might tell their doctor they would be happy just to sit through an entire movie without having to rush to the bathroom. Other women might say they don't mind using pads as long as the leaking isn't too bad and they can avoid surgery. Still other women might say, "Do whatever it takes. I want to laugh and play with my grandchildren and I don't want to wear pads."

Ask your doctor, based on the findings, how realistic he or she feels your expectations are. Remember that treatment for urinary incontinence and pelvic floor disorders takes time, and at this early stage it may be too soon for your doctor to know the complete answer to this and many of the other questions you may have. Do ask questions, but be prepared for the fact that some questions, such as how fast your continence will improve or what you can expect as a long-range outlook for your condition, are not always answerable.

How Much Information Do You Want?

Some patients are naturally interested in getting more information about their medical conditions and treatments. Other patients are simply not comfortable with, or interested in, knowing many details about their body and how their treatments work. Similarly, some doctors tend to give their patients more or less information than others. You should feel free to let your doctor know if you want more or less information than he or she is providing.

Clarify Your Understanding of Instructions

It is essential that you understand the instructions the doctor gives you. One of the best ways to do this is to briefly restate your understanding of each item to the doctor. This allows your doctor to know if you need more or different explanations.

Taking a moment or two to make brief notes prevents you from having to call back the next day for follow-up explanations on things such as how to fill out your bladder diary. Be careful that your note taking does not get in the way of listening carefully to your doctor.

During your appointment, review your understanding of the purpose and dosage for medications your doctor prescribes. For example, if your doctor prescribes a drug for urinary urgency, ask how often you should take the medicine and for how long. This prepares you to notice and ask about any differences between what your doctor and pharmacist tell you about your medications.

Follow-Up Appointments and Second Opinions

A follow-up appointment is an important part of your treatment process. When returning, bring a brief list of any questions or concerns that have come up since your last visit. Your doctor will be interested in detailed and specific information about any changes in your symptoms.

Getting a second opinion (another medical consultation) is another reason why women may see another doctor. In this situation, either you or your doctor believes that getting another physician's perspective is a good way to confirm a diagnosis or a treatment decision. Because doing this helps you get the most effective care, many health insurance policies cover the costs of at least one additional medical consultation.

You can ask the doctor you are seeing or your primary doctor for their recommendations. Another option is simply asking your doctor's nurse for names. If your physician is the one who suggested the second opinion, then he or she will provide names without your having to ask and may even schedule an appointment for you.

Sometimes, with your permission, the two doctors exchange information before the consultation and discuss your case afterward. In many situations, you return to your original doctor for treatment.

MANY HEALTH PROFESSIONALS: MANY PERSPECTIVES

As you will learn in chapter 6, bladder control treatment can involve several types of healthcare providers, each looking at your symptoms, condition, and treatment from a unique point of view. These different perspectives may involve a stronger focus on a specific aspect such as structural anatomy, brain-bladder communication, diet, or childbirth history. You may notice that your bladder control healthcare providers have different viewpoints, vocabulary, and office environments.

The facilities you may go to for various evaluations and treatments may look and feel surprisingly different. For example, some physical therapy facilities are laid out in an open, informal way. Of course, physical therapy offices also have private rooms for the types of treatments that bladder control patients receive to improve pelvic muscle tone! While you will learn about these and other treatments in chapter 8, it is important to keep in mind that you may encounter different types of healthcare providers and treatment settings.

Working along with your doctor, the nurses, physician's assistants, diagnostic technicians, nurse midwives, and physical therapists are among many of the allied healthcare professionals you may see. All are valuable resources. These allied healthcare providers often schedule longer appointments and have more time for follow-up work. This can help you get the treatment and information you need under relaxed conditions.

COMMUNICATION CHALLENGES

An open exchange of information between a patient and her doctor is vital to effective medical care. Your doctor needs to gain a clear understanding of your health history, symptoms, and goals for improvement. This helps your doctor provide you with the best care. Likewise, you are entitled to receive understandable information from your doctor.

Some patients find communicating with doctors difficult. Often this is because both the doctor and the patient feel pressed for time. Sometimes it is simply because the doctor and patient have different ways of speaking and listening. For example, a very soft-spoken and shy patient may find it challenging to communicate easily with a doctor who has a strong, outspoken personal style.

Similarly, a patient who has a very animated way of interacting may feel a doctor who has quiet or methodical mannerisms is not paying attention to her.

In some cases it is the doctor who should adjust her communication approach. However, it is your responsibility to let your doctor know that she needs to change how she talks with you. Otherwise, it probably will not happen! In other cases, to improve the quality of communication, patients need to modify how they interact with their doctor.

Other common medical care communication challenges include embarrassment, cultural and personal style differences, gender issues, language barriers, and medical terminology. Usually, patients can overcome these challenges by using the following guidelines to help get the most from their medical appointments:

1. Bring a list of symptoms and questions
2. Tell the nurse about your medical condition before the doctor comes in
3. Remember that you and your doctor are partners in your care
4. Ask specific, on-topic questions if you do not understand what the doctor says
5. Refer to your list during the beginning, middle, and end of your visit

Limited Time with Your Doctor

When a doctor enters the exam room, both the patient and the doctor can almost hear an imaginary stopwatch start running. The unfortunate reality is that medical office schedules require doctors to keep their appointments limited to fixed-time allocations. This is why it is so important for you to be open and specific when talking with your doctor. Although you must accept the reality of your doctor's appointment schedule, remember that you should have enough time to explain your symptoms and to discuss your treatment options.

An excellent way to ensure the best use of your appointment is to come prepared with a list of bladder control issues you want to talk about. You can divide the list into two sections—one with symptoms and one with questions. Once you are in your doctor's office, use this list to help you focus the discussion and to prevent you from forgetting to mention important symptoms or questions.

Telling the nurse about your medical concerns before the doctor comes in is another helpful strategy. When you do this, the nurse will make notes on your chart or may also mention your concerns to the doctor. This helps the doctor know right away what the appointment will be about. The nurse is also a good resource if you have questions about what may happen during and after your appointment.

Often, patients have several different medical conditions they want to discuss in an appointment. When this is the case, be sure to let the receptionist know when you call for an appointment. Typically, appointments are set up in time slots that may range from fifteen to forty-five minutes. With this in mind, you can tell the receptionist that you have several things to discuss and that you would appreciate having a longer appointment. Usually, "first appointments" are longer ones.

Make a list of your health concerns and prioritize the items. Then, at the start of your appointment, name them off quickly so you and your doctor can decide together which items are most important. Remember that your doctor cannot address a very long list of varied health concerns during a typical appointment. Having the list as a reference, however, will help the doctor decide to schedule another time to cover remaining issues or concerns.

When patients have more than one medical problem to talk about and no list to guide them, they may put off their most frightening or emotionally charged concern until the appointment is almost—or is—over. Doctors know all too well that this "doorknob complaint," coming just as they open the door to leave the exam room, may be a medical condition the patient was too reluctant to bring up earlier.

Asking questions in the right way is another way to make the most of your time with your doctor. Do not wait until the end of the appointment to ask questions about concepts or medical terms. If you do, you may miss out on key information because basic elements of the doctor's explanations were not clear to you.

However, asking too many questions—or asking them at the wrong time—may distract your doctor from efficiently evaluating your condition. Make sure that your questions are specific and focused directly on what the doctor is explaining at that time. Also, try not to interrupt your doctor's train of thought. Give your doctor a chance to finish a main idea or group of instructions before you ask a question or seek an explanation of a medical term.

Sometimes, questions you may have about your bladder control problems and treatment process simply cannot be answered until the doctor has learned more about your condition. Be patient, and keep a list of these questions. They may be excellent discussion points for a follow-up visit or for a referral appointment with another healthcare provider.

Embarrassment

There are many personal reasons why it can feel awkward to discuss bladder control or pelvic organ prolapse problems with a doctor. One of the most common reasons is vocabulary. At first you may need to get used to hearing and using words such as "vagina" or "urinate." Use the glossary in this book to familiarize yourself with the terms used to talk about urinary incontinence. Try to get comfortable with these words by saying them aloud in private. One surprising advantage of using the medical vocabulary is that it can help make an uncomfortable topic feel less personal!

Perhaps you prefer to use the more common word for something, for example, saying "pee" instead of "urinate." That is okay! Your doctor will probably continue using the medical terminology. This is, after all, the language they have used comfortably for many years, both in medical school and in their practice.

The private nature of the pelvic exam or having unfamiliar tests done that involve your genital area can make many women feel uneasy. If the examination gown does not fit well, you can ask for an extra one so you can feel more adequately covered during the exam or diagnostic procedure. It is customary for a nurse to join you and your doctor in the room during a pelvic exam or procedure.

If the anticipation of having a pelvic exam causes you to feel tense, there are steps you can take to reduce this feeling. Arriving early and bringing along something enjoyable to read while you wait in the exam room is often helpful. Taking a deep cleansing breath just before the doctor begins the pelvic examination is another stress-reducing strategy. Think about something else, or chat with your doctor about something light or amusing during the exam. Remind yourself that your doctor is a professional and has trained for many years to do this job. Also remember that you and your doctor are partners in your care.

If you feel uneasy about talking to your doctor, tell the nurse who brings you into the exam room. Just bringing up the subject with the nurse will help you adjust to talking about it out loud. This also gives the nurse a chance to note your feelings on your chart so the doctor can be better prepared to help you talk about your condition. Usually, patients are relieved to find that talking about incontinence is not difficult to discuss in the privacy of the exam room.

Language Issues

Sometimes, doctors or their patients have added difficulty communicating because one—or even both—speaks English as a second language.

If your doctor speaks with an accent that you have trouble understanding, it is appropriate to politely ask him or her to talk more slowly. Usually, slower speech makes a different accent easier to understand. Likewise, if your doctor has difficulty understanding your accent, you need to make similar speech adjustments.

Remember, sometimes when people are nervous or frustrated they speak faster, louder, and less clearly! In many medical facilities, patients who believe language barriers will make talking to or understanding their doctor difficult may ask for a translator. Additionally, many practices advertise in their phonebook listings the languages spoken in their office.

Patients who have hearing loss must let their doctor know. That way, their doctor will know to speak loudly enough, or write down detailed instructions. This ensures that hard-of-hearing patients fully understand what the doctor tells them about their condition, as well as any instructions regarding medicines, danger signs, and preparations for medical procedures. If you are very hard of hearing, it may be wise to bring someone along who can listen with you as a backup.

Cultural and Personal Differences

It is human nature to feel more comfortable with people who are like ourselves. In the United States, doctors and patients come together from many backgrounds. Even when language issues are not a factor, communication styles from one culture to another can be surprisingly different. Of course, doctors are trained to be sensitive to the needs of patients with respect to cultural diversity. Patients, however, may need to be flexible and open-minded when working with a doctor who is from another country or culture, or whose personal style and mannerisms are unfamiliar to them.

Gender Issues

Some women would rather talk with a woman doctor about "female" health issues such as bladder control and pelvic floor problems. However, depending on the doctors working in your area and the providers available through your health insurance plan, you may not have this option. Therefore, remember that providers who treat women's health issues receive the same training regardless of their gender. Rather than limiting yourself to finding a woman doctor, focus on the importance of getting skilled medical treatment for improving bladder control.

GETTING THE SUPPORT YOU NEED

Sometimes, people are simply not comfortable with their doctor but do not have other healthcare provider options. This can happen for many reasons, including limited access to providers because of location, health plan requirements, or financial constraints. Some patients have strong feelings of discomfort in any medical setting. In these cases and others, patients can take steps to help improve their situation. If you believe communication problems will affect your treatment, adopt some other coping options such as bringing along a family member or close friend, or seeking the assistance of a medical social worker that some clinics and hospitals provide for their patients.

A Second Pair of Ears

If you feel you may have difficulty communicating efficiently with your doctor, bring someone you trust to your appointments. Having a friend or family member along can be a calming influence. Before making this decision, make sure:

- You will feel comfortable talking about private issues in their presence
- Your friend or relative will be available to join you for follow-up appointments
- This person will support you with your needs and wishes in mind
- You can count on this person to be on time, reliable, courteous, and respectful of your privacy

Make the most of having a support person with you by having them take notes so you can focus on what your doctor is saying. It is a good idea to review these notes with your support person shortly after the appointment. Doing this gives you a chance to refresh your memory about your appointment and to make sure you can read their handwriting.

Medical social workers and/or patient advocates may be available to patients in larger medical facilities. These support professionals are employed by the healthcare facility to provide free, compassionate, and unbiased practical assistance to patients. The following are a few examples:

- Providing easy-to-understand explanations about patients' health conditions and treatment options
- Helping patients work through health coverage issues with insurers
- Offering patients' families, caregivers, and employers explanations of their medical needs
- Providing information about other health resources

You can ask your doctor, nurse, or medical receptionist about the availability of a medical social worker or patient advocate.

What About Finding a Different Doctor?

Imagine, after having several doctor appointments, you find yourself thinking, "Okay—this just isn't working." Maybe the office is hard to get to, you have to wait too long to schedule an appointment, or you feel this doctor just isn't interested in helping you. If you want another doctor, you are entitled to make that change. Urinary incontinence treatment takes time, so it is worthwhile to have a physician you trust and with whom you can work comfortably.

Some patients are reluctant to talk to the doctor about this because they don't want to seem offensive or impolite. Do not worry. Doctors know there are many reasons (e.g., such as office location and personality differences) why patients make office changes. Although changing doctors for certain reasons may be practical, it is never appropriate for a patient to visit a string of doctors simply to "shop" for a particular diagnosis or treatment option. Remember, you and your doctor are a team and it takes time to learn how to best work together.

Under these circumstances, asking friends about the doctors they like, or using an Internet physician locator Web site to find information about other doctors in your area are all good approaches. Medical association referrals and physician locator services are also helpful resources. In addition, phone book yellow pages list doctors by their specialty.

Whenever you go to a different medical facility, it is your responsibility to have your medical records transferred. To do this you will need to sign a release form or write a request letter. In some cases, a doctor's office will give you your records to carry to the new doctor. Other offices will mail or fax records. If the doctor's office handles the medical record transferal, be sure to call before your scheduled appointment to make sure your records arrive before you do! Doing this will help your new or consulting doctor evaluate you.

At Home and at Work: Talking About Your Condition and Treatment

Your family needs to know how your bladder control problems affect your quality of life. They also need to hear about your treatment process. It may take a little getting used to, but you can begin by talking about your condition as part of normal conversation. This will help your family understand why you want to make another bathroom stop, are reluctant to participate in some activities, or why you are buying absorbency products.

When it comes to treatment, it is very helpful to tell family members when and why you are going to the doctor. Then, later, they can ask how it went or you can tell them what comes next. If no one brings the topic up, then by all means, go ahead and do so yourself! Perhaps you can tell your family the highlights of what your doctor told you. Certainly your family will ask questions that lead to more discussion.

If urinary incontinence symptoms are causing difficulties at work, talk with immediate coworkers, human resource managers, and supervisors about the situation. Talking about urinary incontinence at work may not be easy, but remember that loss of bladder control is a medical condition. You are entitled to a work setting that accommodates your needs so you can do your job well. You may also discover that other women you work with—including your supervisor—may be coping with similar problems! In fact, bringing up the subject at work may benefit another employee who has not had the courage to do so.

While you are receiving treatment, ask your supervisor to give you adequate access to a restroom, as well as a work schedule that allows for doctor appointments. Keep your employer posted as your treatment progresses and your needs change.

RESOURCES FOR BLADDER CONTROL INFORMATION

You do not have to navigate your bladder control treatment process by yourself! In addition to the information your doctor provides, you have many resources that range from local support groups to information available over the Internet. Appendix A of this book provides contact information for numerous resources that provide information and support. Additionally, appendix B offers suggestions for supplementary reading on the topic of bladder control.

Local Resources

Check with local hospitals and larger medical clinics to find out if they offer bladder control information sessions or support groups. Ask your doctor as well—he or she may know of bladder control information or support sources you can turn to. If you live near a teaching hospital, the medical library is another source of information. A librarian can help you begin your search. If you are a senior citizen or one who cares for a senior, contact your local senior community organization as another avenue for local support and information. A local retail medical supplier may be another good resource. In addition to telling you about helpful products, they may also have support group contact information.

If you cannot find a local bladder control support group, consider starting your own! You can find out how to do this by reading the "Take Control Support Group Kit" located on the National Association for Continence (NAFC) Web site (http://www.nafc .org) (see appendix A). You have learned that one in three women in America has urinary incontinence at one time or another, so look around you! Getting a support group together could be as easy as telling a few friends and asking each of them to tell some of their friends. Being part of a support group is a great way to learn about bladder control treatment providers and facilities in your area. Additionally, support groups give you the chance to enjoy camaraderie and hear firsthand about helpful resources, products, and tips that have been beneficial to other participants.

Internet Resources

It seems there is no end to the information available via the Internet. So much, in fact, that it can be a challenge to find legitimate, unbiased, accurate, and up-to-date information. As with many things, the Internet is a "buyer-beware" zone. Carefully consider the source and date of any information you find. Sites produced by government health agencies, university specialty clinics, professional organizations, or nonprofit organizations are often excellent sources of reliable information. Appendix A contains contact information for many such organizations, including the National Association for Continence (NAFC), the American Urogynecologic Society, the National Women's Health and Information Center (NWHIC) of the US Department of Health and Human Services, and the Mayo Clinic.

When searching the Internet, you will discover that many sites are developed and maintained by pharmaceutical companies or other companies with an interest in selling their products. Many such sponsored sites contain helpful information and illustrations. However, remember that sponsored sites often emphasize their own products and services and neglect to mention the benefits of other treatments.

Logos or statements that identify a Web site's affiliations, certifications, quality assurance, usability awards, and sponsorship are usually found at the bottom or either side of Web site "home" pages. Health on the Net Foundation (HON) is an example of an organization that provides accreditation. Web sites meeting this international group's stringent criteria for integrity feature the "HONcode accredited" logo icon. Government-sponsored Web sites such as the National Women's Health and Information Center (NWHIC) (from the US Department of Health and Human Services Office on Women's Health) are reputable sites although they may not be HONcode accredited. In addition, you can usually be confident that an Internet site is a reliable source of information if you can answer "yes" to the following questions about it:

- Is information on the site provided by qualified medical professionals?
- Does the site clearly identify its ownership and all of its affiliations with for-profit and not-for-profit organizations?
- Are commercial products and services presented on the site clearly shown as such?

- Can you find the organization's contact information, Webmaster link, and most recent modification date?
- Does the site specify that the information it contains is not intended to replace the care or advice that your physician provides?

While finding reliable sites is one kind of challenge, discovering the information you need is another. The table below offers just a small sampling of search "keywords" you can use within a search engine such as Google or Yahoo to direct you to bladder control information (table 5.1). Additionally, these keywords can be useful tools once you have found a helpful site to explore. Most Web site "home" pages provide a "search" field box. Typing specific keywords into this search box will direct you to more specific information contained in the site.

Appendix A lists some well-respected organizations whose purpose is to educate the public and support those with urinary incontinence. You may also want to explore and participate in the "chat rooms" accessed through some of these respected sites. Chat rooms can be a good way to "talk" with other women about their control management and treatment experiences. Because Web site addresses are subject to change, we are providing the organizations' name in addition to their Web site address in the appendix. Entering these names in an Internet search engine will direct you to their official Web sites.

MOVING FORWARD

You have learned how effective communication with your doctor

Table 5.1. Examples of Some Helpful Internet Keywords

- Bladder control
- Incontinence
- Kegel exercise
- Menopause
- Overactive bladder
- Pelvic floor exercises
- Stress incontinence
- Urge incontinence
- Urinary incontinence

and exploring various resources can help you improve your bladder control. Now, you are ready to begin the process of teaming with your doctor in diagnosing your condition. Chapter 6 will walk you through the diagnosis process, detailing many different methods your doctor may use to evaluate your condition.

FREQUENTLY ASKED QUESTIONS

1. What if my doctor is nice, but doesn't seem to understand women's bladder control problems?

Talk to your doctor! Tell your doctor how poor bladder control affects your quality of life. Remind them that one out of three women have bladder control problems sometime during their lifetime. You might even have to educate the doctor. If your doctor still is resistant to learning, listening, or providing treatment—ask to be referred to someone with more experience in treating bladder control problems.

2. What should I do if my doctor does not take my problem seriously?

You are entitled to respectful and compassionate care for your health concerns. If for any reason your doctor cannot or will not provide such care, by all means ask for a referral or change doctors!

3. If my doctor does not suggest I see a physical therapist, can I ask for help with pelvic floor exercises?

Tell your doctor that you are not sure if you are doing pelvic floor exercises correctly. Your doctor can evaluate this during your physical exam and, if necessary, refer you to physical therapy.

4. At my health clinic, I never see the same doctor twice. How can I get consistent care?

Good communication is especially important in this situation. Although it may seem like you have to say the same thing over and over again—doing so will help you get appropriate care and make progress. Seeing a medical specialist or an allied health professional, such as a nurse practitioner, within these large practices is another way to get more consistent care.

CHAPTER 6

YOUR DIAGNOSIS

A PROCESS, NOT A QUICK ANSWER

*"In the right physician's office,
it is easy to talk about incontinence."*
Lois—after her first urinary incontinence
evaluation appointment

TURNING POINTS

When you have a sore throat and fever, a painful shoulder, or a hacking cough you cannot wait to talk to your doctor. However, even during an annual gynecological exam, few women ever volunteer that they are having bladder control problems. Maybe the doctor does not ask the right questions, or maybe you quietly choose not to answer them. The reasons why it is easy to seek help for a painful shoulder but difficult to talk about incontinence are both simple and complex at the same time.

Even Lois, quoted above, freely admits that during the eight years she tried to manage her bladder problems on her own, she never asked her primary care doctor for advice. So, after all those years, what happened that made her decide to find the "right physician"?

For her, it was the combination of going to a hospital for another problem and then reading in the local newspaper that the doctor who treated her was also an incontinence expert. Before that, Lois believed incontinence was just something you lived with.

Now, after her first appointment and armed with bladder diary and scheduled urination exercise information, Lois feels confident and hopeful. She wants you to know "this all sounds very doable."

For Mary, her "turning point" was quitting her job to avoid the embarrassment caused by incontinence. For the five years before leaving her job, she felt she was managing stress incontinence well enough. "Now I poop and pee at the same time and I don't even know it. It's a mess and I stay in the bathroom forever cleaning up." Unlike many women, Mary did talk to her primary care doctor about her ongoing and then worsening problems. Now that she wants to do something about it, her doctor has referred her to a women's continence clinic for evaluation and treatment.

For other women unacceptable lifestyle changes, family pressure or encouragement, or a "last straw" embarrassing moment are the turning points that create a strong desire for personal control and dignity. Each woman who makes the decision to seek medical help has her own turning point story.

ANOTHER BIG STEP

After reading the preceding chapters, you should now have a different perspective on urinary incontinence. You know about urinary incontinence risk factors, the "hows and whys" of bladder and sphincter function, the importance of having strong pelvic floor muscles, and strategies that make talking to your doctor easier and more efficient. Even more importantly, you know that incontinence is treatable.

You may have found relief in some of our suggested "first step" home remedies. Maybe bladder diaries and pelvic floor exercises were not helpful or not helpful enough to you. Or, perhaps just discovering that many women who struggle with incontinence do regain bladder control has given you the courage to make an appointment to see your family doctor or gynecologist. Whatever your situation, it is a good idea to talk to your doctor about your bladder control problems. This gives your doctor the opportunity to evaluate your overall health, check for other problems that may also cause or aggravate incontinence, and fine-tune your urge and stress incontinence treatments.

In this chapter you will learn how doctors evaluate and diagnose urinary incontinence. You will also read about the various medical tests your doctor may recommend. The results of these tests help your physician unravel the cause(s) of your condition and determine the best way to proceed with treatment. Learning about these clinical procedures will reduce your "test anxiety" and help you make educated treatment decisions.

Your First Appointment

You may make your first appointment with a family doctor, gynecologist, urologist, or with a specialist such as a urogynecologist, or a *urologist* who has advanced training in female urology. Often your healthcare plan requires that you first see a primary care doctor. However, many health policies allow women to see providers such as a gynecologist or urogynecologist within their insurance network without a referral.

Choose the doctor you feel the most comfortable with. Be sure to bring your completed chapter 4 Voiding Diary and Scheduled Urination Exercises worksheets (pp. 101 and 106) to the appointment. Having these tools at hand will make it easier for you to talk to your doctor about bladder control. Additionally, the information the tools reveal can help your doctor learn more about your symptoms, and may provide insight for an appropriate treatment starting point.

Your first appointment will include a detailed medical history and a physical examination. During the medical history the doctor may ask you about things that range from pregnancy and childbirth experiences to dietary and smoking habits. Urinalysis, to check for a bladder infection, as well as tests that measure your ability to empty your bladder are important parts of the physical exam. Completing Worksheet 6A, "Preparing for Your First Appointment" (p. 159) will help organize your thoughts and questions in advance.

During the physical examination, your doctor looks for physical signs that may explain your urinary incontinence symptoms. This exam includes a thorough examination of your abdomen, urogenital areas, and rectum to check for indications of reduced muscle tone and *neurological* causes for incontinence. Testing your blood or urine in the clinical laboratory may help uncover conditions such as a urinary tract infection that can cause incontinence or complicate its diagnosis.

FIGURING OUT THE PROBLEM

By reviewing patient history and physical exam clues, the doctor can now recommend specific tests to pinpoint the reasons for your bladder control problems. Test results provide the evidence that helps your physician make a diagnosis and develop a treatment plan. Doing this allows your doctor to correlate your medical history and physical examination findings.

Many women feel nervous about the medical tests their doctors have them take. Many of these tests have long, hard-to-pronounce names that instantly make them sound frightening and potentially painful. Afterward, most women say that undergoing the urodynamic and bladder stress tests that you will read about shortly was not anywhere as bad as they expected. Asking questions both improves understanding and reduces anxiety. Worksheet 6B (p. 164) provides a list of questions to help guide pretest discussions with your healthcare provider. Going over this list before your appointment will help you get the information you need.

Describing Bladder Control Problems

The voiding diary that you learned about in chapter 4 is a very important diagnostic tool. Recording your bathroom habits, physical activities, and the beverages you consume for the three days before your appointment helps you and your doctor associate daily activities with leakage and urgency. In addition to the voiding diary information, also record the number of absorbent pads you use each day and the number of times that bladder accidents necessitate a clothing change. Doing this simple, at-home exercise helps your doctor understand what you mean by leaking "lots" or "all the time."

Some women note improvement in their bladder symptoms by just filling out the voiding diary. You might think that something as simple as filling out a form would not do much for a complex problem like incontinence, but as Frances discovered in the beginning of chapter 4, consciously recording your voiding pattern can uncover easily changed habits and behaviors.

Urinalysis

Urinalysis is another important diagnostic tool that can tell your doctor if a urinary tract infection or diabetes is causing or contributing to your bladder control problems. This makes it an especially valuable test for women who are just beginning to seek treatment for their incontinence difficulties.

Screening your urine sample for *bacteria*, *glucose*, and other substances can show if a urinary tract infection, diabetes, or kidney disease plays a role in making bladder control difficult for you (table 6.1). The screening test involves nothing more than handing the nurse a urine sample. The nurse uses a dipstick—a plastic-backed paper strip that contains testing chemicals—to test your urine. When dipped in urine, dipstick chemicals react with substances in the urine and change color. Comparing the dipstick colors to those on a chart tells the nurse if your urine contains sub-

Table 6.1. Common Urine Dipstick Tests	
Test Substance	**Significance**
Glucose	High amounts of glucose in urine may indicate diabetes, thyroid disorders, and kidney disease.
Ketones	Normally absent in urine. Ketones in urine indicate a high-fat and low-carbohydrate diet, diabetes, starvation, prolonged vomiting, fever or hyperthyroidism.
Protein	Exercise and fever can lead to increased protein in urine. Increased protein may also indicate kidney disease and diabetes.
Nitrates	Indicates the presence of Gram-negative bacteria.
Leukocyte esterase	Indicates the presence of white blood cells and a urinary tract infection.
Bilirubin/Urobilinogen	A normal hemoglobin breakdown product. Excessive amounts indicate potential of hepatitis and other liver diseases.
Hemoglobin/Blood	Indicates presence of blood, indicates possible injury, trauma, infection, or urinary tract obstruction due to stones or tumors.

stances associated with having diabetes or a urinary tract infection (figs. 6.1a and 6.1b).

If the dipstick shows you have glucose in your urine, your doctor may want to test you further for diabetes. If nitrates and substances that indicate disease-fighting *white blood cells* are present, you may receive treatment for a bladder infection. To make sure you receive the most effective antibiotic treatment, the nurse will send your urine sample to the clinical laboratory to identify the bacteria causing the infection. This information helps the doctor prescribe the most appropriate antibiotic (table 6.2).

Fig. 6.1. Dipstick urine screening test

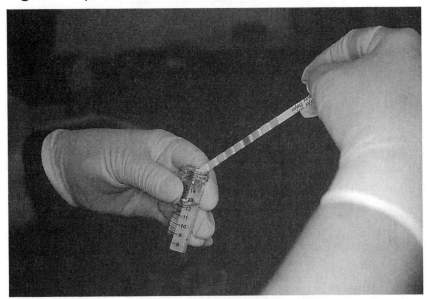

a. Dipping the dipstick into a urine sample

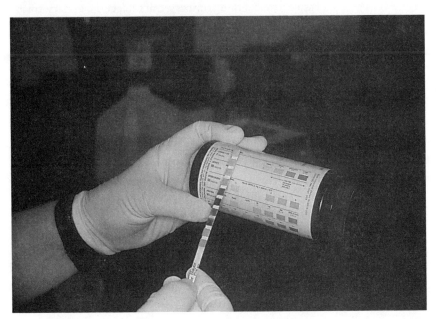

b. Comparing the results to a "normal" standard

Table 6.2. Urine Evaluation

Chemical Characteristic	Some Clinical Implications
pH	In the context of other clinical information, may indicate: Acid: diabetes, infection, starvation Alkaline: infection, vomiting, kidney failure
Protein	Higher than normal values—excessive exercise, kidney disease, infection, trauma, urinary tract obstructions, tumors may increase the amount of protein in your urine
Glucose	Normally we do not have sugar in our urine. Having sugar in your urine can indicate a high sugar diet, diabetes, thyroid disease, advanced kidney failure
Bilirubin	A positive result may indicate hepatitis, liver disease, exposure to toxic agents
Ketones	A positive result reflects a high fat diet, restricted carbohydrates, diabetes, fasting, vomiting
Occult Blood	Normally we do not have blood in our urine. A positive result may indicate a urinary tract infection, urinary tract stones, excessive exercise, hypertension
Calcium	Higher than normal values: mobilization of calcium from bone, hyperparathyroidism, hypercalcuria, bladder and breast tumors Decreased values: vitamin D deficiency, kidney failure
Uric acid	Higher than normal values: gout, viral hepatitis, sickle cell anemia Decreased values: chronic kidney disease, folic acid deficiency, lead toxicity
Magnesium	Higher than normal values: high blood alcohol Decreased values: malabsorption syndrome, chronic alcoholism, kidney disease
Nitrates	Normally we do not have nitrates in our urine. A positive result for nitrates may indicate a bacterial urinary tract infection

Sometimes, treating these problems takes care of the urgency and leaking caused by infection-related inflammation and the large amounts of urine produced as a result of having diabetes. Other times, conditions like diabetes and bladder infections contribute to making overactive bladder and stress incontinence symptoms more difficult for you to manage.

Postvoid Residual

The *postvoid residual* describes how much urine remains in your bladder after voiding. Weak bladder muscles and nerve damage resulting from trauma or diabetes can make complete emptying difficult. Eventually your bladder can become so full that urine overflows and dribbles out, resulting in overflow incontinence.

The *postvoid residual test* measures voiding efficiency. Some facilities use a handheld ultrasound instrument to measure the amount of retained urine after voiding. This procedure is similar to the ultrasound methods used to monitor pregnancies and cardiovascular function.

Preparation for a postvoid ultrasound measurement is very simple. First, to find out how much urine you can void, your doctor or nurse will ask you to urinate into a plastic collection "hat" (fig. 6.2). Then the nurse measures the amount of urine collected.

Next the nurse will ask you to change into an examination gown, or to simply lower your clothing and underwear to reveal your belly. After you lie down on the examination table, the nurse or ultrasound technologist puts a dab of ultrasound gel on your lower abdomen. This gel improves contact between your body and the sound-wave-emitting probe. Then, by moving the probe over your bladder the nurse or ultrasound technologist can read on the monitor screen how much urine your bladder still contains (fig. 6.3).

Removing retained urine with a *catheter* is another way to measure how well your bladder empties. After you have voided, a nurse specialist will ask you to lie down on an examination table as you

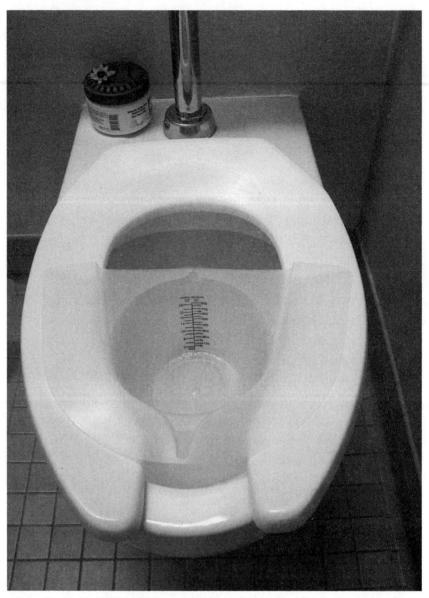

Fig. 6.2. A urine collection "hat" used to measure how much urine you have voided

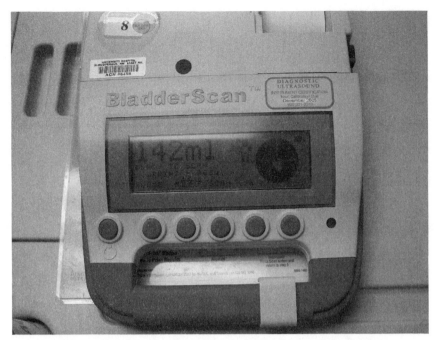

Fig. 6.3. A portable ultrasound unit measures the amount of urine remaining in your bladder after voiding.

do for a Pap smear. Then the nurse will insert a thin, flexible tube or catheter into your urethra and bladder to collect and measure the amount of remaining urine (fig. 6.4). To minimize discomfort, she coats the catheter with an anesthetic gel. You may still feel a slight burning sensation as the catheter moves through your urethra and into your bladder.

Evaluating Your Postvoid Residual Results

A postvoid residual volume of 100 milliliters or less—slightly less than one-half cup—is usually considered normal. However, for many clinicians a postvoid residual of 100 milliliters or anything greater than one-third of the total voided volume requires further evaluation. A single elevated postvoid residual does not confirm a

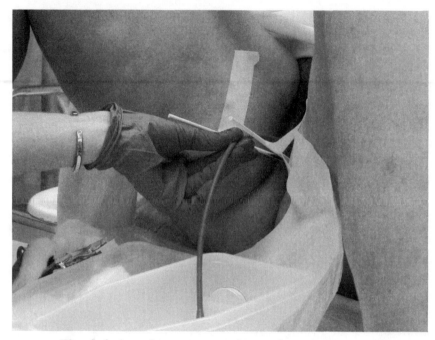

Fig. 6.4. A catheter inserted into the urethra to measure how much urine remains after voiding. Removing retained urine with a catheter is another way to measure how well your bladder empties.

diagnosis of urinary retention. You should receive several elevated postvoid residual measurements to validate this diagnosis. The inability to empty your bladder efficiently may indicate problems that include nerve damage and *pelvic organ prolapse.*

The Bladder Stress Test

The *bladder stress test,* or *simple cystometrogram,* allows your clinician to record your reported urge sensations as your bladder fills with water. Before beginning the test, your doctor or nurse will ask that you go to the bathroom and empty your bladder as you do normally.

Next, the doctor or nurse inserts a catheter through your urethra and into your bladder while you are lying down. Your nurse may also collect some of the urine in a sterile container. This way they also have a sample to test for a urinary tract infection.

So they know exactly how much fluid your bladder can hold, a catheter is used to fill your bladder with a measured amount of sterile, warm water or *saline* solution. Usually this amount is about one-half to one cup of liquid. As this is happening, be sure to tell the technologist or nurse when you first feel bladder pressure and then urgency. Knowing the amount of fluid your bladder can comfortably hold is important information. Then, after removing the catheter, they will tell you to cough.

Coughing places additional pressure on your bladder. As you learned in chapter 3, when this pressure is strong enough to momentarily move your urethra, it may cause a situation where the bladder pressure overcomes urethral pressure. When this happens you may leak urine.

Position is an important factor in getting reliable bladder stress test results. Some women are continent lying down, but because of gravity and the additional pressure exerted by the abdominal organs they are unable to control urine loss if they cough while standing. After filling your bladder, your nurse may ask that you stand and cough.

For a few hours after undergoing this test procedure, you may feel a little soreness when you urinate. Regardless of the discomfort, it is important to drink water and other beverages. Catheterization sometimes introduces into your bladder bacteria that normally live in the urogenital tract. In addition to drinking water to stay well hydrated, taking cranberry tablets to acidify urine and thereby prevent bacterial attachment to the bladder wall may decrease the risk of getting a bladder infection.

Evaluating Your Bladder Stress Test Results

Even with a full bladder, coughing and bearing down should not cause urine to leak from your bladder. If stress incontinence is the reason you leak, the doctor will see a fluid loss right after you cough.

Without coughing, leakage accompanied by urgency may be the result of strong bladder muscle contractions. During the bladder stress test, if you have a bladder contraction, the sudden increase in bladder pressure may push fluid through the catheter and cause leakage. Sometimes, this increase in bladder pressure is strong enough to push the catheter out of your urethra! This combination of symptoms—bladder contractions with leakage—is associated with having overactive bladder.

Cotton-tipped Swab Test

Stress incontinence occurs when the urethral sphincter cannot control the leaking of urine from the bladder. This happens when your urethra moves too much in response to coughing and your bladder pressure is higher than the urethral pressure. Learning how your bladder and urethra move when you cough and bear down helps your doctor provide the most appropriate treatment.

After comfortably situating yourself in the examination stirrups, your doctor or nurse inserts a cotton-tipped swab, lubricated with an anesthetic gel, into your urethra and asks you to cough or strain. Most patients say this test is not painful. However, for twenty-four to thirty-six hours afterward some patients report having a burning sensation that feels similar to having a bladder infection.

Evaluating Your Cotton-tipped Swab Test

The cotton-tipped swab test information tells your doctor whether or not your vagina and pelvic floor supports your urethra. If, with coughing or straining, the swab moves more than thirty degrees from its resting angle, then you have a urethra that moves easily. If the swab does not stray far from its original position, then urethra sphincter weakness may be making bladder control difficult. Often, bladder control problems result from a urethra that is both mobile and not strong enough.

SPECIALIZED TESTING

Although diagnostic procedures such as the bladder stress test and the cotton-tipped swab test are valuable, your doctor may suggest that you undergo more tests. This may happen when your initial tests reveal confusing or conflicting results, or when the doctor suspects something like diabetes is causing urgency and leaking. Presurgical evaluation is another reason you may have to undergo more specialized procedures such as *cystoscopy* and urodynamic testing. Doing this helps your surgeon tailor your bladder surgery to meet your needs.

Looking Inside Your Bladder

Cystoscopy allows the doctor to examine the inside of your urethra and fluid-filled bladder. To do this, a *cystoscope* is used. It is an instrument that consists of a miniature camera, a thin fiber-optic tube, and an intense light source (figs. 6.5a and 6.5b).

Cystoscopy is a safe procedure that doctors usually perform in their office or clinic using local anesthesia. When women have certain painful urinary tract conditions the doctor may opt to do this procedure in an operating room where they have better anesthesia options.

Before undergoing this procedure, you will sign a consent form. Should the need arise, your signature gives the doctor permission to remove a small sample—or *biopsy*—of any suspicious-looking bladder tissue for laboratory evaluation.

You do not need to *fast* if you are going to have a cystoscopy in your doctor's office. If your doctor does the procedure in the operating room you will receive special preparation instructions. Usu-

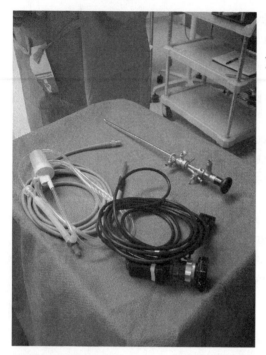

Fig. 6.5a. A cystoscope unit used to look inside your bladder

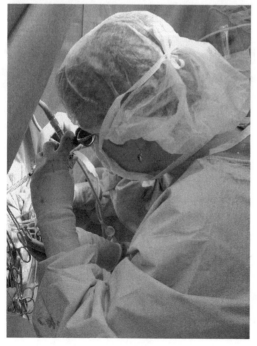

Fig. 6.5b. Using a cysto-scope to look inside the bladder during a surgical procedure

ally these directions involve not eating or drinking after midnight the evening before the cystoscopy.

In either situation, it is important that you inform your doctor or nurse about the medications or herbal treatments you take by mouth. It is especially important that they know if you take medications that affect bleeding such as aspirin and ibuprofen and blood thinners such as warfarin (Coumadin).

Using local anesthesia, you may feel a little discomfort as the cystoscope moves through the urethra and into your bladder. Like the bladder stress test, you may feel urgency when the cystoscope catheter fills your bladder with sterile water or saline. Having a full bladder makes it possible for your doctor to examine the bladder wall surfaces and other structures.

Evaluating Your Cystoscopic Procedure

Viewing the images on the monitor or directly through the cystoscope, the doctor can observe how well the urethra and bladder neck respond to coughing and bearing down. It can also be determined if the ureters, coming from the kidneys, are effectively transporting urine to your bladder. Sometimes kidney stones, growths, or inflammation are found to cause or contribute to your symptoms.

Urodynamics

Urodynamic testing measures pressure differences between your abdomen, bladder, and urethra. These measurements help your doctor understand how your bladder responds to filling, coughing, and bearing down. Urodynamic measurements can also help your surgeon decide which surgical procedure or combination of procedures will give you the best results. Sometimes urodynamic testing will reveal overactive bladder—a condition that is not treated surgically.

Since less complicated methods, such as your incontinence history, bladder stress test, postvoid residual testing, and the cotton-tipped swab test, can help distinguish between stress and overactive bladder symptoms, doctors do not usually include urodynamic testing in their initial workup. Many doctors use urodynamic testing when the previous procedures fail to produce conclusive results, or as part of a presurgical evaluation. Urodynamic testing can help identify other causes of incontinence, such as multiple sclerosis, the aftereffects of strokes, long-term diabetes, and trauma.

Using a catheter to fill your bladder slowly with sterile water or saline mimics what normally happens when your bladder fills with urine. Sensors inside the catheters detect pressure changes and muscle contractions. A computer converts these responses into easily interpreted information that you and your doctor can see on the computer screen.

For this test, you will need to come to the testing facility with a full bladder. Shortly after your arrival, you will be asked to urinate. Rather than using the restroom, you will void in a special portable toilet, similar in appearance to a sickroom commode, to measure the rate at which you urinate. Called a urine/flow study, this part of the urodynamic test determines if an obstruction, such as vaginal prolapse, is causing urgency or urine retention and dribbling. These studies can also reveal flow patterns that may indicate weak bladder muscles.

Although the surroundings are unusual, it is important that you urinate as you normally would in your own bathroom. The doctor and nurse will leave the room at this time.

After urinating, a medical professional uses a urinalysis dipstick to test your urine for signs of having a bladder infection. Urodynamic testing increases the risk of spreading a bladder infection to other parts of your body. A positive dipstick test for bacteria in your urine means you cannot undergo urodynamic testing until you have received treatment for the infection. If the dipstick test is negative for bacteria then the urodynamic test proceeds.

Now that your bladder is empty, you are ready to begin the next part of the test. Like many other gynecological procedures, you position yourself on the examination table and place your feet in stirrups. Next, the doctor or nurse inserts a catheter coated with a lubricating and pain-numbing gel into your bladder. Some patients report a "pinging" feeling as the catheter moves into the bladder.

Using the inserted bladder catheter, your doctor or nurse can remove and measure any remaining urine. This postvoid residual measurement tells them if urinary retention is a problem.

With the bladder catheter in position, another catheter is placed into your vagina or your rectum. This step is sometimes a little uncomfortable. Bearing down as though you are having a bowel movement makes placing an anal catheter easier.

Sensors in these two catheters measure and record muscle contractions and the pressure in your bladder, urethra, and abdomen. These measurements tell your doctor if strong or frequent bladder muscle contractions are making bladder control difficult for you.

Then, similar to the bladder stress test, the doctor slowly fills your bladder with warm water or saline. To help your doctor evaluate the relationship between pressure and bladder muscle behavior you must pay close attention to how your bladder feels as it fills. It is important to report the following sensations when you first experience them:

- Bladder pressure
- Pressure increasing to the point that you would normally think about finding a bathroom
- A strong urge to urinate

This part of the test shows the relationships between bladder filling, urgency sensations, and increases in bladder and urethra pressure.

Urodynamic testing can also show how your bladder and urethra respond to outside pressure such as a cough or *Valsalva* (bearing down). Your doctor or nurse will ask you to give a weak, moderate, and strong cough. Doing this determines the ability of your urethra to resist increases in abdominal pressure. You may be asked to do this test both while reclining and while standing.

A pressure/flow study, with your bladder containing a known amount of fluid, is the final portion of your urodynamic study. Similar to the urine/flow study described earlier, you empty your bladder into the special portable toilet. The sensors, still in place, record how your bladder and urethra respond to voiding.

Urodynamic testing usually takes less than an hour to complete. Afterward, you can drive yourself home or to work. The next time you go to the bathroom you may feel a little soreness. This discomfort will quickly disappear. Some doctors give antibiotics to reduce risk of getting a test-related bladder infection. Drinking water and taking cranberry tablets are also helpful. Studies show that risk for infection after urodynamic testing is very low.

Video Urodynamics

Video urodynamics, a combination of video imaging with urodynamic testing, is another evaluation method. A video is made that shows what actually happens when your bladder, urethra, and sphincters respond to bladder filling, coughing, and bearing down.

Similar to the methods used to detect intestinal problems, a radiologic technologist fills your bladder with *contrast media*. This nontoxic substance makes it possible to use an x-ray screen to see urine moving through your bladder and urethra.

Evaluating Your Urodynamic Results

Urine/flow studies show how fast your bladder empties over a certain amount of time. So, in addition to being interested in how much your bladder holds, your doctor is also looking at voiding patterns.

Making a graph of how fast urine leaves your body provides a voiding pattern picture. When everything is working properly, urine first comes out slowly, then rapidly increases in rate and then slows down again until you are empty. If you have a blockage or a weak detrusor muscle, then urine leaves your bladder slowly and it takes a long time before you are either empty or you stop urinating.

Filling your bladder with warm water or saline allows your doctor to record and determine two important bladder characteristics:

1. The amount of fluid your bladder can comfortably hold
2. Bladder stretching characteristics

Normally, you will experience strong urge feelings when your bladder contains approximately one to two cups of fluid. Women who struggle with overactive bladder symptoms may experience contractions and strong urge sensations with less than one cup of water in their bladder.

Muscle activity sensors within the catheter help clinicians distinguish between stress incontinence and leaks resulting from an overactive bladder. Leakage *without* bladder contractions indicates stress incontinence. Leaks *with* bladder contractions may indicate overactive bladder.

Sometimes—even though coughing, sneezing, and bladder contractions make you lose urine at home—this does not happen during your urodynamic testing session. Obviously, this does not mean that you do not have bladder control problems! In this situation, your doctor must always be careful to evaluate your urodynamic test results in the context of your patient history, signs, symptoms, and other diagnostic tests.

With the sensors in place, pressure/flow studies can reveal the weak or irregular bladder contractions typical of having multiple sclerosis or other neurological problems. The many small ups and downs on the graph help illustrate what kind of problem you may have.

Unlike the bladder stress test, urodynamic studies produce numerical or quantitative data. This means that in addition to having evidence to support a diagnosis, your doctor also knows the actual bladder pressure that causes you to lose urine.

For some women, even small bladder pressure differences cause bladder control problems. Other women, because of compensating conditions or behaviors, only leak when the pressure is very high. Knowing how well or how poorly your sphincter resists bladder pressure may be an important treatment consideration.

WHAT COMES NEXT?

After undergoing some or even all of these tests, your doctor will evaluate the results and then discuss various treatment options with you. Even though you may have already kept a voiding diary, made dietary changes, and spent time working on pelvic floor and scheduled urination exercises, your doctor may want you to work on these things a little while longer. Although this may make you feel impatient, it is important to give these relatively simple, safe, and noninvasive treatment options a chance to work.

Sometimes your test results show that something other than urgency or stress incontinence, such as a weak detrusor muscle, incomplete emptying, or poor coordination between your bladder and urethra, is making bladder control difficult for you. In chapter 7, you will learn how pelvic organ prolapse, a condition where the pelvic floor cannot adequately support the vagina, bladder, and uterus, is another important bladder control factor.

Many women are surprised to discover that surgery is not the only treatment option for urinary incontinence. Other ways to manage or reduce incontinence include wearing an internal pelvic organ support pessary, taking medications to reduce the frequency and strength of bladder muscle contractions and—believe it or not—physical therapy. You will learn more about these safe and noninvasive treatment strategies in chapter 8.

WORKSHEETS

Worksheet 6A: Preparing for Your First Appointment

Taking a detailed medical history and performing a thorough physical exam is how your doctor begins the diagnosis process. Completing and bringing a copy of this questionnaire to your appointment will make it easier for you to provide important information.

The Problem

How many months/years ago did you first notice problems with urine leakage? _____ months _____ years

Has it gotten worse since you first noticed it? (circle one) Yes / No

About how many times during each day do you go to the bathroom to urinate? _____ times

How many times do you get up each night to go to the bathroom? _____ times

Do you feel that you have to run to the bathroom to get there in time? (circle one) Yes / No

Do you ever lose urine before getting to the bathroom? (circle one) Yes / No

How often do you lose urine? (circle one) More than once a day, once a day, once a week, rarely

Describe how you lose urine. (check all that apply)

Is it a dribble? _____ Is it a gush? _____

List the type of activities, such as coughing or standing up, that cause you to lose urine: _____

_____

After you urinate, does it still feel like you have to go more? (circle one) Yes / No

When on the toilet, is it difficult for you to start the flow of urine? (circle one) Yes / No

When you urinate, is the stream a dribble? (circle one) Yes / No

When you urinate, is the stream a forceful stream? (circle one) Yes / No

Do you wet the bed at night? (circle one) Yes / No

Do you ever have blood in your urine? (circle one) Yes / No

Is urinating painful? (circle one) Yes / No

Everyday Habits

Do you wear absorbent pads? (circle one) Yes / No

If yes to the above question, how many pads do you use a day? _____ pads

Does leaking cause you to change your clothes? (circle one) Yes / No

Approximately how much fluid (all beverages) do you drink each day? (write the number of ounces) _____
Do you drink caffeinated beverages? (circle one) Yes / No
Do you drink coffee? (circle one) Yes / No
Tea? (circle one) Yes / No
Colas? (circle one) Yes / No
Do you drink alcoholic beverages on a daily basis? (circle one) Yes / No
Do you smoke? (circle one) Yes / No

Medical Conditions

List your major surgeries and their dates.

Surgery	Date
A.	
B.	
C.	
D.	
E.	

Do you have diabetes (high blood sugar)? (circle one) Yes / No

Do you have hypertension (high blood pressure)? (circle one) Yes / No

Pregnancy

How many pregnancies have you had? (give number) _____

How much did your largest baby weigh? _____ pounds _____ ounces

Did any of your deliveries require any cutting and stitching? (circle one) Yes / No

Did you have any forceps-assisted deliveries? (circle one) Yes / No

Did you have any vacuum-assisted deliveries? (circle one) Yes / No

How many of your deliveries were cesarean births? (give number) _____

Bladder Infections

Do you have frequent bladder infections? (circle one) Yes / No

How many bladder infections do you have each year? (give number)
_____

Do you ever experience pain or a burning sensation during urination? (circle one) Yes / No

Have you noticed an unusual color to your urine? (circle one) Yes / No (describe the color) _____

Have you noticed an unusual odor to your urine? (circle one) Yes / No (describe the odor) _____

Medications

List all the medications you currently take. Include vitamins and herbals.

A. Prescription medicines:

Medication	Dose	How often taken	How long have you been taking the medicine?

B. Over-the-counter medicines and vitamins and herbals:

Medication	Dose	How often do you take it?	How long have you been taking the medicine?	Why do you take this medicine?

Worksheet 6B: Some Questions to Ask Your Provider Before Taking a Medical Test

What is the name of the test?
Why do I need this test?
How will the test result affect my diagnosis or treatment?
How much does this test cost?
What are the risks associated with taking this test?
Are there less risky or less costly tests?
What is the likelihood of getting inaccurate results?
How do I prepare for this test? Do I need to restrict:
  Food?
  Water or other beverages?
  Alcohol?
  Or reschedule medications?
  Exercise or other activities?
What are the consequences if I delay or do not take this test?
If I need to take several tests:
  Which are the most important tests?
  Is there an advantage to taking them all at one time?
  Can we schedule the most important tests first?
When will you get results?
What do the results mean?
What is the next step if the results are normal?
What is the next step if the results are abnormal?

Before taking a test you should make your doctor aware if you have concerns about:

  Costs
  Insurance
  Fears regarding the test itself

It is also important that your doctor know about:

The medications, herbal treatments, and vitamin supplements that you normally take.

Any medical conditions that might interfere with test results or your ability to take the test.

Any previous test results.

FREQUENTLY ASKED QUESTIONS

1. What if my doctor does not ask me questions about things that I believe may have some bearing on my bladder control problem?

In the course of your exam the doctor should provide opportunities for you to express your ideas. However, by providing complete and descriptive answers you can often create these important opportunities. For example, your doctor will most certainly ask you if you have difficulty controlling your urine flow. Rather than limiting your answer to yes or no, be sure to say "Yes, but it is very painful when I urinate" or "No, I don't have a problem controlling urine flow. What is hard for me is getting all of it out." By providing complete answers, you help your doctor make a realistic diagnosis and may even save yourself the added time and expense of getting unnecessary tests and inappropriate treatment.

2. Can any doctor provide all these tests?

Your primary care doctor or general-practice gynecologist can do postvoid residual and bladder stress testing. Not all primary care doctors have the equipment and the expertise to do other types of testing, so you may need to find a facility that specializes in diagnosing and treating urinary tract problems. Often these are specialized group practices located within larger medical centers or private group practices.

3. How can I find a specialized practice where I can get one-stop help?

Your primary care physician and your gynecologist can make suggestions and referrals. If your primary care physician or gynecologist doesn't do it, you can also find these specialists in the phone book yellow pages listed under headings such as "urogynecology," "urology," "women's health," and "gynecology." Other resources include the professional specialty and organization lists provided in chapter 5.

4. Do these tests hurt?

Most women report that these tests are not nearly as painful as they sound. The anesthetic and lubricating gel reduces catheter placement discomfort. Rather than painful, many women use words such as "uncomfortable," "odd-feeling," and "strange" to describe how they felt while undergoing these diagnostic procedures. As with many things, consciously relaxing your body makes it easier to cope with unfamiliar surroundings and unusual body sensations.

CHAPTER 7

RELATED PROBLEMS

PELVIC ORGAN PROLAPSE
AND ANAL INCONTINENCE

*"When this bulge began to fall out of my
vagina, I was worried that I had cancer."*
Beverly—in relief, after her pelvic organ prolapse evaluation

WHAT IN THE WORLD IS THIS?

Shirley, a fifty-year-old busy mother of four, was worried. Something was wrong "down there" and whatever it was—it was getting larger. "Could it be a tumor?" she wondered. "Or maybe," she thought, "this is one of those never-talked-about menopausal changes."

She remembered the bladder control problems she had after her last pregnancy nearly fifteen years ago. It was a difficult delivery and soon afterward, Shirley couldn't cough or sneeze without wetting herself. However, the many years of religiously doing the pelvic floor exercises her obstetrician had recommended made bladder control something she rarely thought about. Shirley wondered if this troubling new situation was related to what happened earlier.

The bulge—whatever it was—didn't hurt and didn't bleed. It also seemed to get bigger on those days when she was on her feet all day at work. While sitting on the toilet or lying in bed, Shirley found she could easily push the bulge back inside. But as soon as she stood up, it slid out again.

Over the months the bulge got bigger and the leaking stopped. In fact, Shirley was alarmed that she couldn't urinate without first pushing the bulge back inside her body. Even with all the inconvenience and discomfort, it was another year before Shirley got the courage to make an appointment and ask her gynecologist, "What in the world could this be?"

PELVIC ORGAN PROLAPSE

You might be thinking, "I know I leak urine, but what I have seems different from what my friends say about their leaking problems." Urinary incontinence is often accompanied by other pelvic floor problems including *pelvic organ prolapse* and *anal incontinence*. Many of the same reasons women develop urinary incontinence can also contribute to these other problems (fig. 7.1).

Pelvic organ prolapse happens when pelvic floor attachments and muscles are no longer in their proper positions and sag. This causes the vagina, and the pelvic organs behind it, to fall toward or even slide out through the vaginal opening. Once the vagina is no longer inside the body, the pelvic organs lose the support the vagina normally provides and they follow the same downward path. However, you do not actually see your pelvic organs because they are covered by a layer of vaginal skin! This is similar to a hernia that occurs elsewhere in the body. Abdominal hernias cause the contents of the abdomen to protrude, like a bubble, between the abdominal wall muscles, but remain covered by skin. Pelvic organ prolapse causes the pelvic organs to protrude from the vagina in a similar manner.

You know you have a prolapse when you feel or see tissue pro-

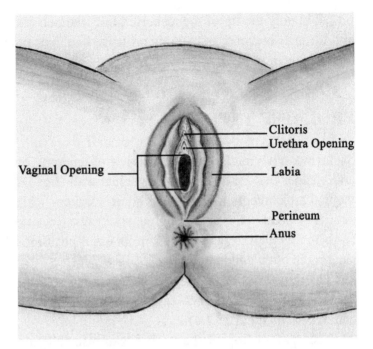

Fig. 7.1. A drawing of a woman's normal external genitals, showing the normal relationship between the vagina and anus

truding from your vagina. Sometimes symptoms are subtle and can include feeling pressure or pelvic discomfort. You may notice that your symptoms worsen in the afternoon or after physical activity. This is because standing and physical activity put additional pressure on your pelvic organs and pelvic floor.

Of course, other serious problems, including cancer, can cause a growth to appear in your genital area. If you notice something protruding from your vagina, it is important to have a medical professional evaluate what the bulge is.

How often prolapse occurs is unknown. Approximately one in eight women will eventually have surgery for urinary incontinence, pelvic organ prolapse, or both problems. However, this number is probably only the tip of the iceberg. Many women are like Shirley and do not seek care until their prolapse becomes uncomfortable and interferes with daily activities.

PROLAPSE TYPES

So far we have focused our discussion of anatomy on the urethra and bladder that lie on the upper vaginal wall (fig. 7.2). When the vaginal attachments to the pelvic bones weaken—causing them to stretch or break—the upper vaginal wall sags. Because the bladder rests on this wall, it also falls from its usual position. This kind of sagging is often called a *cystocele* (fig. 7.3).

The same kind of sagging can occur in the bottom vaginal wall that sits over the rectum. A sagging bottom vaginal wall is often called a *rectocele* (fig. 7.4).

The *apex*, or top of the vagina, can also fall from its normal position and may even slide down and out of the vaginal opening. Sometimes the uterus, located above the vaginal apex, also falls along with the vagina. Though many believe otherwise, the uterus does not cause the prolapse—it is simply following the prolapse out of the body. Even if you have had a hysterectomy (the removal of your uterus), the vaginal apex can still sag and slide out. With or without the uterus, this type of prolapse causes the vagina to turn inside out like a pants pocket. *Enterocele* is the common term for this type of sagging (fig. 7.5). Often women have pelvic support weaknesses that include all three regions of the vagina.

You may also have other problems that are directly and indirectly related to having a weak pelvic floor. Stretching of the vaginal opening happens when the pelvic floor muscles are not strong enough to keep the vagina closed. Thinning of the *perineum* or the tissue between the vaginal and rectal openings is another problem.

Often prolapses are not as severe as the ones just described.

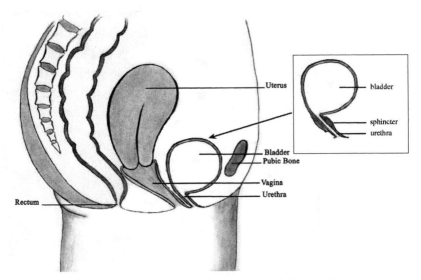

Fig. 7.2. Normal position of the pelvic organs.

Although the pelvic organs may not be 100 percent in place, they do not sag enough to produce noticeable or bothersome symptoms. A prolapse that remains inside the vagina, rarely, if ever, requires treatment. On the other hand, sometimes even a mild or small prolapse may cause noticeable symptoms such as pelvic pressure or lower back pain. Big or small—if your prolapse is bothersome or causes discomfort, you should go to your doctor for evaluation and treatment.

WHAT IS IT LIKE TO HAVE
PELVIC ORGAN PROLAPSE?

Most women find it difficult to describe the often vague and nonspecific symptoms typical of prolapse. The most common complaint of severe prolapse is the statement: "It feels like I am sitting on a ball." Women also mention pelvic pressure, low back pain, as well as con-

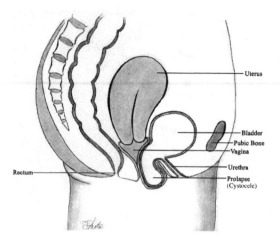

Fig. 7.3. Cystocele—prolapse of the bladder through the upper vaginal wall. The uterus and rectum are in their normal positions.

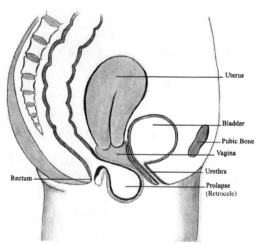

Fig. 7.4. Rectocele—prolapse of the rectum through the back vaginal wall. The uterus and bladder are in their normal positions.

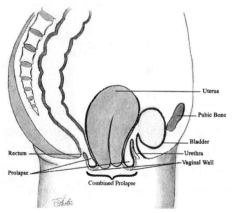

Fig. 7.5. Enterocele with rectocele—prolapse of the uterus, bladder, and rectum, which have all fallen from their normal positions and the vagina has turned inside out.

stipation and difficultly emptying the bladder. Patients may feel like the stool gets "stuck" even though it is of normal consistency.

Some women have to push the bulge back inside to urinate or have a bowel movement. Do not be embarrassed to tell your doctor that you have to use your fingers to push the bulge inside. This important clue helps your doctor evaluate your prolapse.

Prolapse usually occurs gradually, although it may seem to change suddenly when the bulge protrudes from your body. Although you might think that it would hurt to have your vagina turned inside out, few women say it is painful.

If you have a prolapse that involves the upper vaginal wall, you may have trouble emptying your bladder. This is because the ure-thra, as it and/or the bladder falls downward, may become kinked and block urine flow. Figure 7.3 illustrates a case in which the bladder wall is falling downward.

Overactive bladder is another problem that can come with having severe pelvic organ prolapse. The pressure of the prolapse forces the bladder to work especially hard to empty, which can cause bladder muscles to contract even when the bladder is not full. Some women find that they cannot void or may have to take a very long time to empty their bladder. As you can imagine, these are very uncomfortable situations.

Constipation is another common problem for women who have prolapse. However, unlike "dry and hard" constipation, these women report having soft stools that feel "stuck." Although this may sound strange, they are describing what happens when the lower vaginal wall sags and no longer supports the rectum. Without proper support, stool cannot easily pass through the anus.

A large prolapse, over time, can cause stretching damage to the nerves and muscles of the bladder, vagina, and rectum. The good news is that once you receive prolapse treatment, nerve and muscle function may improve, leading to better bowel and bladder function. The possibility of preventing long-term damage is a good reason to seek medical help. You can use Worksheet 7A located at the end of this chapter to help identify your prolapse symptoms and any anal incontinence symptoms you may also have. You will learn about anal incontinence and how it is related to pelvic organ prolapse later in this chapter.

EVALUATING YOUR PROLAPSE

Your physical exam findings (see chapter 6) help your doctor diagnose and evaluate pelvic organ prolapse. After taking a patient history, your healthcare provider will ask you to get undressed and lie on an exam table as though you were having a Pap test.

Doctors have several ways to describe prolapse size and severity. Many doctors will tell their patients that they have a first-, second-, or third-degree prolapse. This roughly corresponds to having a small, medium, or large prolapse. Other doctors use a ruler to measure the vaginal protrusion. The hymen, located at the vaginal opening, is the reference point. If you hear a negative number, this means your prolapse is still inside your body and does not protrude past the hymen. If you hear a positive number—like +4—this means your prolapse has fallen outside of your body. However, you probably already knew that! (See table 7.1; figs. 7.6 and 7.7)

Some doctors describe prolapse using standardized *staging* categories. Rather than just describing a prolapse as small or big, staging also takes into consideration what part of the vagina is sagging. The stages, numbered from 1 to 4, refer to the prolapse severity. A stage 4 prolapse is bigger and more advanced than a stage 2 prolapse.

During the examination, your doctor may ask you to cough or Valsalva to see how far the vagina protrudes with additional abdominal pressure. Then, similar to your Pap test exam, your doctor uses a *speculum* to open the vagina. Doing this allows healthcare professionals to look at your cervix as well as inspect and measure the length of your vagina. Next, your doctor will place

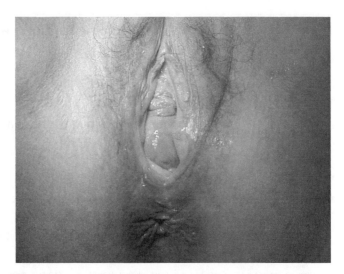

Fig. 7.6. This prolapse, several centimeters out beyond the hymen, is a +2.

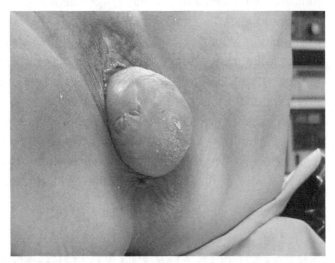

Fig. 7.7. An example of a very large prolapse at +8 centimeters beyond the hymen. The vagina is turned inside out.

Table 7.1. Bladder Prolapse Measurement	
Number	**Prolapse Position**
-3	Normal position
-2	Beyond its normal position but does not sag very far
-1	Almost to the hymen
0	To the hymen
+1	Only slightly beyond the hymen
+2	Several centimeters beyond the hymen
+3	Many centimeters beyond the hymen
+4 or higher	Very far past the hymen, to the point that the vagina may be nearly completely inside out

half a speculum against one wall of your vagina and ask you, once again, to Valsalva. Repeating this for each side, your doctor will look for evidence of upper and lower vaginal wall sagging as well as vaginal apex sagging (figs. 7.8a and 7.8b). At the end of this examination, your doctor may ask you to either stand in place or sit on the toilet to make the vagina protrude as far as possible. Since the severity of the prolapse can vary with activity or time of day—it is important that your doctor see the prolapse at its worst.

Your doctor will also measure the upper and bottom walls and top regions of the vagina, as well as the sizes of the vaginal opening and perineum. These important measurements help your physician describe your prolapse using standardized terminology and to plan the best way to treat it.

TREATMENTS FOR PELVIC ORGAN PROLAPSE

There are only three things you can do about pelvic organ prolapse. First, if the prolapse is small and not bothersome, you can wait and see if your condition changes. Should this happen, and the prolapse

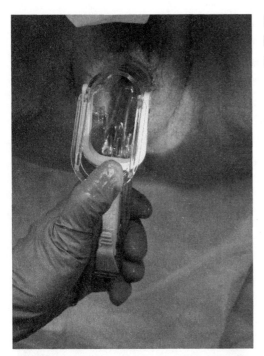

Fig. 7.8a. A speculum helps the doctor look inside your vagina.

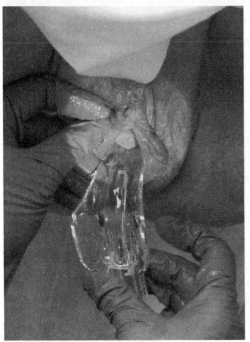

Fig. 7.8b. Next, your doctor will place half a speculum against one wall of your vagina. This makes it possible to see if there is prolapse on the other side. In this example, the protrusion of tissue above the speculum indicates an upper wall prolapse, or cystocele.

becomes troubling or begins to noticeably protrude, make an appointment with your doctor to discuss treatment options.

Second, if the prolapse is causing you discomfort or other problems, you can use a removable pelvic organ support ring or *pessary*. You will learn more about pessaries in chapter 8.

The third treatment option is surgery. Because there are many ways to treat pelvic organ prolapse surgically, your surgeon will rely on your physical exam results to decide which procedure, or combination of procedures, is right for you.

What is the success rate of prolapse surgery? Well, that depends on your definition of success. And as you can imagine, doctors and medical researchers have a difficult time defining success. Some gauge treatment success by "reduced symptoms" such as less discomfort or reduced incontinence—and others say "improved patient anatomy," meaning improved pelvic organ support. Time is another success factor. Is a successful surgery one that lasts one year, five years, or forever?

However you decide to define success, in reality as many as one in three women find their prolapse symptoms return within twelve years after their surgery. This statistic should not dissuade you from considering surgical repairs. For many women, having many years of improved function is worthwhile. When prolapse surgery does "fail," women may have the option to have another surgery. You can improve your odds for getting a lasting or "good" surgical repair by doing a little research. You will learn more about what constitutes a "good" surgical procedure in chapter 9.

Most people assume that having surgery will restore the bladder and bowel function they once had. Unfortunately, this is not true. Certainly surgery can correct structural problems such as reattaching the vagina to the pelvic bone, but doing this does not always restore or even improve continence. Surgery cannot repair the damaged nerves and muscles that control your bladder and bowel. When nerve and muscle damage is not extensive, surgery may eventually improve function.

ANOTHER HIDDEN PROBLEM

Jane, a retired schoolteacher, stopped going to church because she was embarrassed. At first the embarrassing problem occurred infrequently, but recently it had happened more and more often. Her first sign was the smell. A quick check in the restroom confirmed her worst fears— she had leaked stool into her underwear without even knowing it.

Some of her friends mentioned having "bladder difficulties" but none of them had even whispered about having this problem! Because of the smell, it was very hard to hide or manage this kind of incontinence. She felt as though she was never really completely clean, and rather than risk an accident in public, she stopped socializing altogether.

ANAL INCONTINENCE

Anal incontinence, the involuntary loss of gas or fecal material, occurs in up to one in three women who have urinary incontinence. Doctors evaluate anal incontinence severity based on frequency and type of fecal loss. Involuntary passing of gas usually occurs first. Later, this may progress to the inability to control watery stools and then solid or formed stool. Gas is the most difficult bowel material to control, followed by liquid and solid types of fecal materials. However, it is important to remember that *anyone* who has severe diarrhea may also have temporary anal incontinence.

The occasional loss of gas may not be troublesome or call for treatment. In fact, nearly everybody can admit to having gas problems at one time or another! If frequent loss of gas prevents you from doing your job, being intimate, or socializing then you may want to consider treatment.

Fecal incontinence is emotionally devastating. This means that anal incontinence is rarely discussed among family and friends, or between patients and their doctors. The good news is that many of the treatments used to improve urinary incontinence: pelvic floor exercises and increased fluid and fiber can also help many women control anal incontinence.

What Causes Anal Incontinence?

Causes of anal incontinence include anal sphincter damage, chronic diarrhea, or chronic constipation with stool impaction. Perineal tears resulting from childbirth are probably the most common cause of anal incontinence.

To understand how anal sphincter damage causes anal incontinence problems, we first need to know how things normally work. It is tempting to think of our digestive or *gastrointestinal* system as a tube with a plug in the end. If the plug doesn't work, you leak stool. As is almost always the case, things are not quite so simple. Anal continence is the result of complex interactions between the gastrointestinal tract and the pelvic floor nerves and muscles.

How Does Anal Continence Work?

The gastrointestinal tract ends with the anal sphincter complex that includes the *internal anal sphincter*, the *external anal sphincter*, and a cushion of tissue rich in blood vessels. It is these vessels that sometimes develop into painful and itching hemorrhoids. These three structures encircle the rectum and keep it closed. The internal sphincter does the lion's share of the moment-to-moment continence, while the external sphincter contracts when a cough or sneeze places extra stress on the continence mechanism.

The pelvic floor muscles, particularly the *puborectalis muscle*, also play an important role in maintaining anal continence. The puborectalis is a sling of muscle that stretches from the pubic bone to behind the rectum. When contracted, it helps to form a "kink" and prevents the passage of stool (fig. 7.9).

When gas, liquid, or formed stools arrive at the anus, "sensory

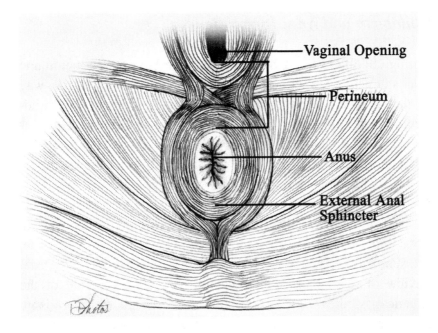

Vaginal Opening

Perineum

Anus

External Anal
Sphincter

Fig. 7.9. The external anal sphincter and muscles of the pelvic floor are responsible for maintaining anal continence.

sampling" allows the anus to make an appropriate decision. Specialized sensory organs tell the anal sphincter that it is time to pass gas (if we have a moment of privacy) or to wait until later if it senses fecal material. This messaging between the brain and the anus is similar to how the brain-bladder connection works. Because the anus can recognize and distinguish between gases, liquids, and solids, some say that the anus is the smartest muscle in the body!

This system can have problems making the right decision when severe diarrhea overwhelms the sphincter complex or nerve damage prevents detection. When this happens, the sphincters may not respond correctly to sensory information and fail to contract in time.

Childbirth and Anal Incontinence

During childbirth, the baby's head can tear both the perineum and anal sphincter. Sometimes these tears can extend all the way through the anal sphincter and into the rectum. Usually such childbirth-related injuries are repaired at the time of delivery. Unfortunately, even though your doctor did a good job of putting the sphincters back together, there may be lasting nerve or muscle damage. This may keep things from working as well as they once did. Sometimes the sphincter pulls apart, even after repair.

A surgical cut, or an *episiotomy,* is sometimes performed during labor to prevent (in theory) ragged tearing and the nerve, muscle, and sphincter damage that can lead to problems later on. Not true! Review of research results presented in a recent Journal of the American Medical Association publication reveals that there is no proven benefit of performing routine episiotomies during childbirth. Some severe childbirth tears occur under the perineal skin where they are invisible to the unaided eye. By using the same ultrasound techniques used to see an unborn baby, clinical researchers find that as many as one in three women who have a vaginal delivery may have a hidden tear. Fortunately, even if a vaginal birth damages the anal sphincter, it does not always lead to anal incontinence. This is because other muscles, like the puborectalis, can pick up the slack.

The Anal Incontinence Examination

If you have anal incontinence, speak to your doctor or nurse about it. Keeping anal incontinence "hidden" by avoiding social interactions does not solve the problem. Even if your doctor does not ask you about this problem, use some of the suggestions in chapter 5 to initiate this conversation. Getting a medical referral to a gastroenterologist, urogynecologist, or colorectal surgeon to evaluate and treat your symptoms will help you regain your dignity and quality of life.

To evaluate anal incontinence, your doctor will take a thorough history including what type of material you lose—gas, liquid, or solid stool—and how often this occurs. Your doctor may ask if you wear a pad to protect your clothing and whether fecal loss affects your social life. Your doctor will also perform a pelvic exam to check for prolapse and a rectal exam to look for other causes of anal incontinence.

The rectal exam usually involves a visual inspection of the anus and the perineum to look for things such as hemorrhoids, infections, scars, and other conditions that might cause anal incontinence difficulties. Similar to testing for stress incontinence and vaginal prolapse, your doctor may ask you to bear down to see if you have a prolapse.

To check for neurological function your doctor will stroke the perineal skin. Normally, doing this causes the anal sphincter to contract and pucker into the easily observed "anal wink." A lack of response indicates that nerve damage may be the cause for your anal incontinence problems.

An anal exam is the last part of your rectal exam. With a gloved and lubricated finger your doctor will evaluate your anal canal. Doing this allows the physician to judge anal sphincter tightness, and with a voluntary pelvic floor muscle contraction, the ability of your anal sphincter and puborectalis muscle to tighten and maintain continence. This tactile examination, with and without Valsalva, allows your doctor to feel for scars and rectal masses.

Anal Incontinence Tests

Similar to making objective measurement of bladder function, your doctor may ask you to have tests to:

- Measure how well your anal sphincter works
- Determine whether or not you have an anal sphincter tear
- Evaluate the neurological function of your anus

While the rectal exam can tell your doctor if you have a weak or strong anal sphincter, it does not provide information about how a sphincter injury or function affects continence. Some of the tests used to assess anal incontinence include:

- Anorectal manometry—a painless ten-minute procedure that measures anal sphincter resting tone and squeeze pressure.
- Anorectal electromyography—a twenty-minute procedure during which your doctor uses very small needles to evaluate communication between nerves and the anal sphincter.
- Ultrasonography—a test that uses a small anal probe to take a 360-degree ultrasound picture of the internal and external anal sphincters.

Other specialized tests for anal incontinence include:

- Colonoscopy—a test that uses a fiberoptic tube that is advanced into the rectum to determine if the rest of the rectum and colon is healthy and free from disease such as inflammatory bowel disease or cancer.
- Defecography—a radiological test where the rectum is filled with a paste similar in consistency to stool. X-rays are taken while you bear down, cough, squeeze your pelvic floor muscles, and defecate to see how well the pelvic floor works as a unit.

This may seem like a long menu of procedures. But not all doctors perform all tests on all patients. Your doctor will talk with you about which of these procedures are most appropriate for your situation. Remember to ask any questions you have about the nature of the tests, their importance, what the doctor hopes to find, and how the finding will relate to your incontinence.

TREATING ANAL INCONTINENCE

Similar to managing urinary incontinence, management strategies that involve diet changes, pelvic floor exercises, physical therapy, or certain medications can help you control anal incontinence. Although it will take time and patience before you see results, many specialists recommend that you try these methods before considering surgical repairs. Anal continence, in addition to requiring intact tissues, also involves complicated nerve-muscle interactions. Because surgery does not restore nerve function, the likelihood of long-term anal continence improvement in women who have severe nerve damage is low.

Treatments Using Medical Management

Increasing dietary fiber is the usual first-step treatment for anal incontinence. Dietary fiber improves anal continence by helping you produce soft, bulky stools that the anal sphincter can easily sense and respond to. Using the tips in chapter 4 as your guide, gradually increase dietary fiber to prevent gas and flatulence.

The pelvic floor exercises discussed and described in chapter 4, in addition to helping you control overactive bladder and stress incontinence symptoms, also strengthen your anal sphincters and puborectalis. Without question, pelvic floor exercises are a great investment of your time and energy!

Your doctor may also suggest that you see a physical therapist who treats pelvic floor problems. Similar to the physical therapy treatments you will read about in chapter 8, these physical therapists have procedures to specifically help improve anal continence. One of these treatments, biofeedback, retrains the rectum to detect the presence of stool. To do this, therapists use a probe similar to the type used to measure anal pressure.

Sometimes, the best management strategy for anal incontinence is medications, such as loperamide (Imodium) that cause constipation. Combining constipating drugs with scheduled *enemas* helps prevent the involuntary loss of feces. Table 7.2 lists medications commonly used to treat anal incontinence.

Surgery and Anal Incontinence

The mainstay of surgery for anal incontinence is sphincteroplasty, where the anal

Table 7.2. Drugs commonly used for the treatment of anal incontinence
Drug Names
• Loperamide
• Diphenoxylate with atropine
• Hyoscyamine sulfate
• Alosetron
• Cholestyramine

sphincter is sewn back together. Although many women do report having better anal control afterward, this improvement may not last beyond five years. Nonetheless, many women say that they would undergo the surgery once again even for this less than perfect result.

ANOTHER CAUSE FOR INCONTINENCE— FISTULAS

A *fistula* is a hole or a tunnel that develops between two adjoining body cavities. Infections or tissue damage resulting from surgery or poor blood circulation cause many types of fistulas to form. When a hole forms between the bladder and the vagina, urine continually drains through the vagina. In the developed world, fistulas are an uncommon aftereffect of having a hysterectomy, while in developing nations, most fistulas are the result of limited labor and delivery care and prolonged labor. Surgery to close the hole is the only way to treat this type of incontinence.

Sometimes fistulas form between the rectum and the vagina. This type of fistula allows fecal material to drain out from the vagina. This sort of fistula can occur after childbirth, particularly in women with a severe childbirth tear, or after surgery. They can also occur in women who have rectal infections or inflammatory bowel disease. Again, surgery is the only treatment. It is important to inform your doctor about urine or stool that comes out of your vagina so you can receive treatment.

LET'S TALK

Not every woman who has bladder control difficulties also has pelvic organ prolapse or anal incontinence. However, knowing about these conditions makes it easier to talk about them and improves the likelihood of receiving the most effective treatment.

Pelvic organ prolapse can occur along with or contribute to urinary incontinence. In some cases, it is not possible to get relief from one condition without also treating the other. Telling your doctor about constipation, lower back pain, and pelvic pressure—things that you may not ordinarily think to mention along with your urgency or stress incontinence symptoms—is important!

Most women find it difficult to talk about intestinal gas and fecal continence. Even though all of us pass nearly a quart of gas daily, we pretend intestinal gas does not exist. In addition, the words we know to use may sound childish and in some cases even impolite. But when things are not working properly, women lose more than bladder and anal control. Women also lose self-confidence, dignity, and the ability to work and socialize with colleagues, friends, and family. Fecal incontinence can make women feel embarrassed, shamed, and dirty.

In chapter 8, you will learn about nonsurgical bladder control treatment options—how they work, what type of healthcare provider administers them, and what expectations you can have for improvement. Many of these medical treatments, such as pessaries and biofeedback, are also used to treat pelvic organ prolapse and anal incontinence.

WORKSHEETS

Worksheet 7A: My Symptoms

This worksheet may seem familiar to you—you filled out a similar worksheet in chapter 2 to describe your bladder incontinence symptoms and how they affect you. Now you can use this list to identify the anal incontinence or prolapse symptoms you may have and how often you experience them. Use the space provided at the end to describe any other symptoms you have. This worksheet can also be a helpful communication tool—take it with you to your next doctor's appointment.

When I sneeze, cough, or laugh I leak (check all that apply) ____ gas ____ liquid stool ____ solid stool	I feel a bulge coming out of my vagina ____ yes ____ no
My anal leakage occurs: ____ daily ____ weekly ____ monthly ____ rarely	My vaginal bulging is: ____ bothersome to me ____ NOT bothersome to me
My anal leakage is: ____ bothersome to me ____ NOT bothersome to me	To have a bowel movement or to urinate, I need to push in my vaginal bulge: ____ rarely ____ sometimes ____ often
When I have the urge to have a bowel movement, I cannot make it to the restroom on time: ____ rarely ____ sometimes ____ often	I have more feelings of pelvic pressure at the end of the day or when I have been active: ____ yes ____ no

My anal leakage occurs:	The bulge in my vagina makes it difficult for me to have sexual intercourse:
___ daily	
___ weekly	___ rarely
___ monthly	___ sometimes
___ rarely	___ often
I wear pads to help manage anal incontinence:	I have difficulty emptying my bladder
___ daily	___ rarely
___ weekly	___ sometimes
___ monthly	___ often
___ rarely	
I leak stool or gas during sex:	I have a very weak flow of urine
___ rarely	___ rarely
___ sometimes	___ sometimes
___ often	___ often
	My bladder does not feel like it empties completely
	___ rarely
	___ sometimes
	___ often
	I have difficulty emptying my rectum:
	___ rarely
	___ sometimes
	___ often
If you have symptoms in the column above, you may be having anal incontinence.	If you have symptoms in the column above, you may be having pelvic organ prolapse.

If you have symptoms from both columns, you may be having both anal incontinence and pelvic organ prolapse.

Other Symptoms and Information:

My anal incontinence symptoms began:

   ___ slowly

   ___ suddenly

I have been having anal control problems for:

   ___ weeks

   ___ months

   ___ years

   ___ more than ten years

My prolapse symptoms began:

   ___ slowly

   ___ suddenly

I have been having prolapse problems for:

   ___ weeks

   ___ months

   ___ years

   ___ more than ten years

Other symptoms I want to discuss:

_____

_____

_____

_____

_____

_____

_____

_____

_____

_____

FREQUENTLY ASKED QUESTIONS

1. What if I have all three problems—urinary incontinence, pelvic organ prolapse, and anal incontinence? Can all three be treated at the same time?

Often the treatments for urinary incontinence, anal incontinence, and prolapse overlap. For example, pessaries can treat both prolapse and urinary incontinence. Pelvic floor exercises can treat both urinary and anal incontinence. If you plan on surgery, procedures to treat all three problems are commonly performed together.

2. Is pelvic organ prolapse or anal incontinence dangerous?

Pelvic floor disorders such as urinary or anal incontinence and pelvic organ prolapse are not life-threatening conditions. However, they are important to treat because these functional disorders affect your quality of life.

3. I have difficulty emptying my bladder because of prolapse. Will I be able to empty my bladder better after treatment for prolapse?

It is difficult to predict what happens to bowel and bladder function when prolapsed organs are repositioned inside the body. Remember, when the prolapse is "out" the urethra can become kinked, making it difficult to empty your bladder without using your fingers to push the bulge inside your body. Simply removing the kink may not solve the entire problem. To empty, the bladder muscle needs to be healthy enough to squeeze urine out. Women with a long-standing large prolapse may have permanent nerve and muscle damage that impairs the ability of the bladder muscle to squeeze.

4. I used to leak urine a long time ago, but as my prolapse got bigger, the incontinence went away. Why is that?

This is also a result of urethral kinking. As the prolapse increases in size, it can obstruct the urethra, and may result in less leakage while the prolapse is out of your body. When the prolapse is treated the incontinence can return because the "kink" is no longer there. This is like kinking and unkinking a garden hose. When kinked, no water exits the hose. But you can expect a big change when you "unkink" the hose.

5. I have been doing pelvic floor exercises and have increased the fiber in my diet and can now control bowel movements, but I have increased difficulty with flatus. Is there anything that I can take to help with these symptoms?

Beano® or Gas X® are two over-the-counter medications that can help with flatus production. Eating fresh parsley also helps.

6. If I have surgery will it cure my incontinence or prolapse?

Curing pelvic floor disorders depends on what your definition of cure is. Can surgery improve symptoms and quality of life? Yes. Can surgery restore anatomy and function as though the problem never existed? No. Medical researchers find that of women who undergo surgery for their prolapse or incontinence, one in three will need to return for another surgery. This shows that surgery is not always a permanent solution. Most women who have surgery say bladder and bowel function, though improved, is different than when they were much younger. It is important to talk to your surgeon about realistic expectations before you decide to go ahead with surgery.

7. Will a prolapse become more serious without treatment?

Doctors really do not know the answer to this question. No one has done a scientific study where a large group of women were tracked over a prolonged period to see what happens with their prolapse without treatment.

CHAPTER 8

TAKE CONTROL

WITH A LITTLE OUTSIDE HELP

*"It is very liberating not to feel like
a toddler with soggy pants."*
Nancy—happy pessary wearer

WHAT A NICE CHANGE!

L ooking at her you would never know what she had gone through. Linda, after years of taking care of children and managing a family business, will soon have the college degree she started nearly thirty years earlier.

It wasn't always like this. Her last pregnancy changed her life. The delivery was a difficult one, involving an *episiotomy* and vacuum-assistance. Soon after the delivery, she was horrified to discover that she wet herself every time she bent over or squatted. Her doctor said that incontinence after a difficult birth is common and the problem would take care of itself.

Well, it didn't. It just got worse. Her doctor then suggested surgery, but warned her that the improvement may last only a few years. At age forty-three, Linda felt she needed to wait before using this only chance for continence.

For the next eight years she tried to manage severe stress incontinence on her own. She cut disposable baby diapers to fit inside her underwear. She always took a change of clothing with her when she left the house. During the day, she religiously went to the bathroom once every hour to prevent having big accidents. She avoided being intimate with her husband. He did not know the extent of her incontinence problem and she did not want him to find out.

Colds and allergies created extra challenges. "When I had a cold, I just sat on the toilet when the coughing got real bad."

In recalling some of her most difficult times, Linda describes allergy season as "constantly wet season." To make sure an unexpected sneeze did not ruin furniture, she sat on plastic sheets and bathroom towels.

By chance, Linda found a magazine article that explained various techniques doctors now have to treat women's urinary incontinence problems. After reading it she realized that she could do better than coping with cut-up baby diapers. She made an appointment with a local urogynecologist. "I was so psyched! Rather than saying hello, I just said, I want a pessary!"

However, it wasn't that simple. After the patient history and a thorough physical exam, the doctor did several tests to assess Linda's situation. Linda recalls the doctor saying that a pessary might not work, but it was certainly worth a try. Well, it did work! And not only is Linda dry, she is now interviewing for her dream job.

PHYSICAL THERAPY AT HOME

If you are doing the pelvic floor exercises that you learned about in chapter 4, then you are already using physical therapy to help yourself achieve continence. However, the long-term effects of childbirth, diabetes, and other medical conditions can make it difficult for some women to identify and effectively exercise their pelvic floor muscles.

Some women who do not have prolapse find that vaginal weights are a good "at-home" solution for helping identify and effectively exercise these specific muscle groups. You can purchase vaginal weights without a prescription at hospital supply stores, pharmacies, and over the Internet. Most companies box them in sets of five or six that range in weight from slightly less than 1 ounce to nearly 2.5 ounces. Each weight looks like a plastic tampon. Similar to a tampon, you remove the weight by relaxing your vagina and tugging on the attached string.

Using vaginal weights is not difficult. First, insert the lightest weight into your vagina. Then squeeze your vaginal muscles and stand up. If you are doing your pelvic floor exercises correctly the weight stays in place when you squeeze. If it falls out, you are actually flexing other muscle groups or pushing down on your pelvic floor.

Once you learn to squeeze the right muscles, you can start using the weights to strengthen your pelvic floor muscles and possibly reduce your stress incontinence symptoms. Begin by finding the heaviest weight you can hold in your vagina for one minute. Remember to start timing after you stand up.

Do your pelvic floor exercises with this weight twice a day. Gradually increase the time until you can hold the weight in your vagina for fifteen minutes. Continue doing these exercises until you can hold the heaviest weight for fifteen minutes.

While vaginal weights are an effective way to exercise pelvic floor muscles, not every woman can use them. To use weights, you must be able to perform a moderately strong pelvic floor squeeze. If you are pregnant, menstruating, or if you have had recent sexual intercourse—refrain from using vaginal weights until a later time. If you have vaginal prolapse, a urogenital tract infection, or if you have had pelvic surgery within the last three months, discuss the safety or value of using vaginal weights with your healthcare provider.

If you have difficulty using vaginal weights, talk to your doctor or nurse. They may have some helpful tips to offer you or may suggest that you see a physical therapist.

GOING TO THE PHYSICAL THERAPIST

Physical therapy can be an important part of your incontinence treatment program. Physical therapists, like other medical professionals, specialize in treating certain areas of the body. This means the physical therapist helping you regain continence has specialized incontinence or pelvic floor rehabilitation training.

Going to a physical therapist is similar to having an appointment with other healthcare professionals. Some physical therapists work alone or in group practices, and others chose to work as part of a comprehensive healthcare team. In either situation, your physical therapist always communicates with your referring doctor.

Before your appointment, your physical therapist reviews a summary of your patient history, physical exam, and test results. Even though a lot is already known about you, the therapist will take another medical history. This may seem repetitive to you and maybe even annoying. However, it is important that your physical therapist hear responses to these questions in your own words. Doing this gives you the chance to update information and discuss things that may have been overlooked earlier.

In some medical practices, the physical therapist might also be the person who helps you begin your voiding diary and scheduled urination exercises. In other situations, your doctor initiates these treatments and the physical therapist is responsible for following up on your progress.

After your physical therapy session, the therapist informs your doctor about evaluation findings, your improvement, and future treatment recommendations.

PHYSICAL THERAPY AIDS

Pelvic floor exercises, biofeedback, and electrostimulation are three treatments physical therapists commonly provide for incontinence patients. Although your doctor may have already told you about the importance of doing pelvic floor exercises to quiet urgency and to reduce stress incontinence, the physical therapist will check to make sure that you are doing these exercises effectively.

If you are having difficulty doing your pelvic floor exercises, the physical therapist might try biofeedback to help you learn to identify and better control specific muscle groups. In addition, electrostimulation can help reduce urgency caused by an overactive bladder.

Biofeedback

Biofeedback is a term used to describe the responses we make to body and environmental changes. It is something all of us do every day—without even thinking about it. We breathe faster when our body needs more oxygen, we shiver when we are cold, and urge sensations send us to the bathroom. All of these biofeedback examples are ones where signals from our body or our surroundings cause behavior changes.

Biofeedback also includes our responses to the information we get from measuring tools such as the bathroom scale when, after getting brave enough to look, we adjust diet and exercise to compensate for weight gain or loss. We are also making biofeedback adjustments when we take medication to regulate our blood pressure or heartbeat rate.

Another type of biofeedback helps you control what are normally involuntary bodily functions. For example, learning biofeedback techniques can give you voluntary control over processes that are usually involuntary such as regulating your pelvic floor muscles and urinary sphincter. This takes time and patience.

First, the therapist places sensors on your belly to detect abdominal wall contractions and in your vagina to monitor other muscle groups. Connecting the sensors to a computer allows you to see how well you contract and relax various muscles on the computer monitor (fig. 8.1).

Seeing what actually happens as you do pelvic floor exercises helps you to modify these body functions as you contract and relax different muscles. Although at first it is a trial-and-error process, eventually you become skilled at controlling specific muscles. The therapist can also give you helpful suggestions.

Improving your pelvic floor exercises both strengthens the pelvic floor muscles and reduces stress incontinence symptoms.

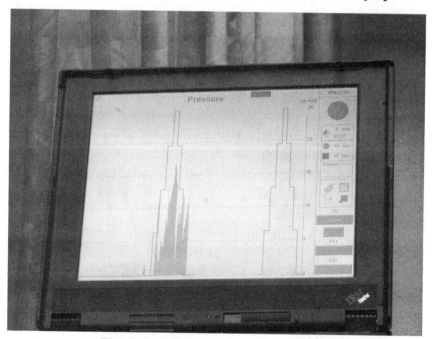

Fig. 8.1. Patients use biofeedback to see how well they are doing their pelvic floor exercises. This patient is learning how to do the elevator exercise pattern. She can see her muscle contractions represented on the monitor.

Effective pelvic floor exercises also help you to control overactive bladder symptoms by reducing urgency sensations.

Revisiting Pelvic Floor Exercises

As you learned in chapter 4, pelvic floor exercises are a way to help women strengthen their pelvic floor muscles, control urgency sensations, and prevent urine leaks resulting from stress incontinence. Like many things that are "easier said than done," doing pelvic floor exercises correctly is sometimes challenging. Some women, because of childbirth injuries or other medical conditions, find it difficult or impossible to isolate and contract this muscle group.

Physical therapy can help you regain the coordination and muscle strength needed to perform pelvic floor exercises efficiently. Combining biofeedback with the quick flick, contract and release and elevator exercise patterns that you learned in chapter 4 is a technique physical therapists use to help you recover muscle coordination and strength.

Electrostimulation

"You are going to do what?" That, according to Kathy, a university hospital physical therapist, is what most patients say either verbally or by raised eyebrows, when she mentions electrostimulation. Electrostimulation is not as bad as it sounds. It is similar to the treatments used to reduce postoperative pain or other muscle discomfort and works by making you less sensitive to nervous system stimulation. Electrostimulation reduces urgency by resetting brain-bladder communication paths.

After you position yourself on an examination table, the physical therapist places a small current-generating probe into your vagina and then hands you a keypad. This means you are in control and can stop treatment if it gets uncomfortable (fig. 8.2).

Electrostimulation treatments usually last for fifteen minutes.

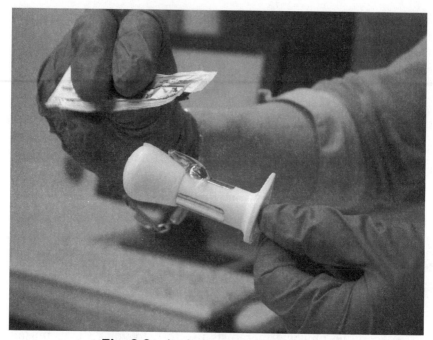

Fig. 8.2. A physical therapist applies a lubricating gel to the current-generating probe used for electrostimulation therapy.

During that time, the machine cycles between delivering ten seconds of low-voltage electricity and fifteen seconds off. Doing this causes your pelvic floor muscles to contract and improves muscle tone. Women typically come in once a week for treatment sessions for a period spanning six to eight weeks.

According to one eighty-five-year-old patient, electrostimulation "feels weird but does not hurt."

PESSARIES

As the old saying goes, "necessity is the mother of invention." Since ancient times women have inserted objects into their vagina to help

Fig. 8.3. Pessaries are not a new treatment. This inflatable rubber ring pessary is nearly one hundred years old! (Gertrude Frishmuth Collection)

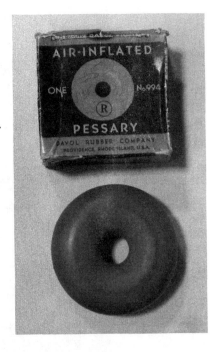

improve continence. Some examples of early makeshift pelvic supports include stones and other objects made from brass, gold, and silver. Today, tampons are a common home-remedy solution for incontinence since they, too, provide vaginal and urethral support.

It took the invention and development of flexible rubber in the mid to late 1800s before manufactured pelvic organ support products were available. One of the first was a doughnut-shaped inflatable rubber ring (fig. 8.3).

Inserting a pelvic organ support or *pessary* into the vagina is a safe and noninvasive way to help manage stress incontinence. Now, instead of using tampons or inflatable rubber rings, women use flexible silicone pessaries to help support pelvic organs and reposition the urethra.

Incontinence pessaries come in a range of sizes and shapes that include rings and dishes (fig. 8.4). Having a wide selection of pessary choices improves the chance that your healthcare provider can find one that will both fit you comfortably and improve continence.

Fig. 8.4.
Incontinence ring pessaries come in many sizes. It may take several tries before you find the one that gives you the best fit.

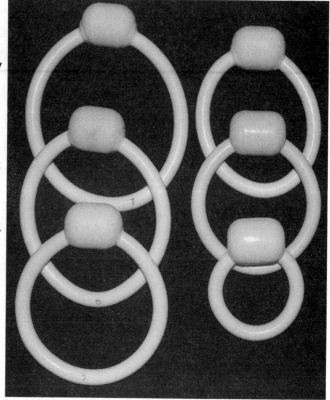

Who Can Wear a Pessary?

Many healthy women use pessaries on a long-term basis as a way to postpone or avoid surgery. Pessaries are also a good solution for those having bladder control problems while pregnant or who are too medically frail to safely undergo surgery. Sometimes women have stress incontinence only while doing strenuous exercise. A pessary is a safe and simple solution for physically active women. Since many pessary styles are easy to insert and remove, some women use them only when jogging, playing soccer, doing aerobics, or even gardening. You should not wear a pessary if you have an active vaginal infection or *pelvic inflammatory disease* (PID). After treating the infection, you may resume wearing your pessary.

Not every woman can successfully wear a pessary. Tissue irritation is a problem for women who are allergic to silicone. Those who have very weak pelvic floor muscles, or who have already undergone pelvic floor surgery may have difficulty keeping the pessary in place, because the vagina is too narrow or scarred to allow for pessary placement.

How Do Pessaries Help?

Like a supportive and cradling hammock, pessaries keep the pelvic cavity organs from sliding downward. Certain pessary shapes are used specifically to manage stress incontinence. These ring-shaped pessaries in figure 8.5 have a knob that slightly compresses the urethra and elevates the bladder neck. This pessary style improves continence by increasing the urethral pressure and normalizes the angle between the bladder and the urethra. Now, when you cough, sneeze, or get up from a chair the pessary helps the urethral pressure remain high enough to withstand increases in abdominal pressure.

Choosing the Right Pessary

Like finding a pair of comfortable shoes, getting fitted for a pessary is a trial-and-error process. First, your provider will select the pessary style that best matches your needs. The incontinence ring pessary is commonly used to alleviate stress incontinence symptoms. Looking like a baby's teething ring, this pessary is nothing more than a flexible silicone ring with a knob that pushes against, supports, and repositions the urethra.

The incontinence ring pessary is also a common solution for exercise-induced stress incontinence. Many clinicians and their patients prefer such a pessary for this purpose because it is comfortable to wear and easy to remove.

For situations where there is also mild prolapse, incontinence dish pessaries are another option. This pessary, in addition to the

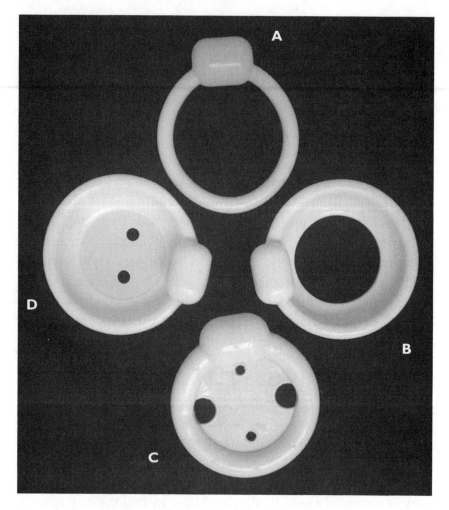

Fig. 8.5. Pessaries commonly used to treat stress incontinence with and without pelvic organ prolapse

A is an incontinence ring pessary used to treat incontinence without pelvic organ prolapse.

B is an incontinence ring pessary with a rim that makes the ring less flexible so it can provide more support for pelvic organs.

C is an incontinence ring with prolapse support.

D is an incontinence dish for mild prolapse.

knob, also includes a support rim or floor that prevents the pelvic cavity organs from sagging into the vagina (fig. 8.5).

Getting the Right Fit

The next consideration is finding the largest pessary that you can comfortably wear. Most ring-shaped pessaries range from just under two inches to slightly more than four inches in diameter. This may seem large to you, but remember, babies also fit in the vagina!

Because there are so many styles and sizes to choose from, pessary fittings take time, patience, and experience. To help make the process more time efficient and cost effective, your doctor or nurse will first fit you with a trial pessary.

After performing a pelvic exam the doctor or a nurse specialist will lubricate, fold, and insert a mid-sized pessary into the vagina. As it moves to the top of the vagina, it unfolds and thereby supports the organs located above it (figs. 8.6, 8.7a-c, and 8.8). Once in place, the examiner will assess the fit. The ability to slide a finger between the pessary and your vaginal wall is a first test. The pessary is too big if a finger cannot easily sweep between the two surfaces and too small if it feels too roomy.

Next the doctor or nurse will test how well the pessary does its job. You will be asked to bear down, cough, and do the kinds of activities that normally cause you to leak. If the pessary both fits comfortably and provides adequate support, you will not leak. A well-fitted pessary should not cause you pain or discomfort. In fact, you should not even feel its presence!

Your doctor will also ask you to go to the bathroom and void. A pessary that is too big may do its job too well and can make urination difficult or even impossible. If this happens, you will be fitted with the next smaller size. Pessaries that are too small, in addition to not helping you, may actually fall out. Having very weak pelvic floor muscles is another reason why pessaries do not stay in place.

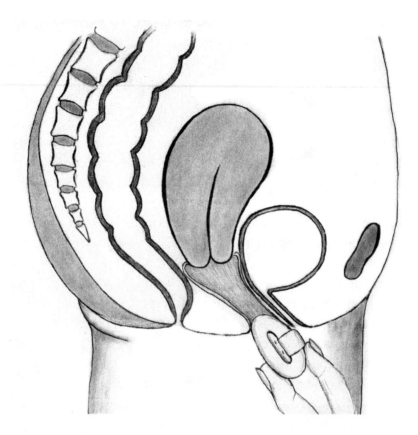

Fig. 8.6. Learning how to insert a pessary is not difficult. First fold the pessary and slide it into the vagina. Then, after it opens, rotate the pessary so the knob points toward your head. This will position the incontinence knob under your urethra.

After finding the right-sized pessary, your doctor will either provide you with an in-stock pessary or order one for you. Most health insurance policies will pay for both your doctor visits and the pessary. A follow-up visit, scheduled after wearing your new pessary for one to two weeks, allows you and your doctor to decide if this is the best pessary for you. Be sure to tell your doctor about any

Fig. 8.7. Here a nurse is showing a patient how to insert a pessary.

a. A dab of estrogen-containing cream helps keep the vaginal tissues healthy.

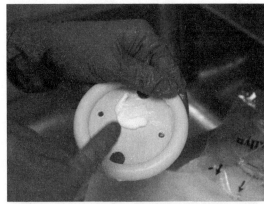

b. Folding the pessary and inserting it into the vagina.

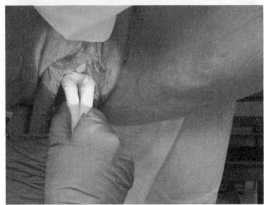

c. Sliding it into place.

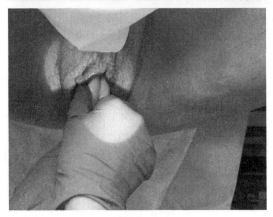

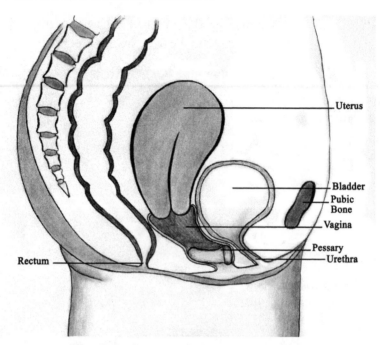

Fig. 8.8. Here is the pessary in place. Note that the knob sits under the urethra. Because the vagina stretches and easily changes shape, sexual intercourse is possible with the pessary in place.

discomfort you may have. Also report any problems with stress leaks and the ability to void or have a bowel movement. Your doctor will do a pelvic exam to make sure the pessary still fits well as well as remove and clean the pessary.

Once fitted, most women can learn to care for their pessaries on their own and remove, clean, and reinsert their pessaries weekly. If patients cannot care for their pessaries themselves, they need to see their doctor every four to six weeks to have their pessaries removed and cleaned. You will read more about pessary care later in this chapter.

Wearing a Pessary

You should be able to comfortably wear your pessary while doing all of your normal activities. A question often asked is: "Can I have sex while wearing a pessary?" As with many things—it depends. However, most incontinence pessaries can stay in place during intercourse.

When you talk to your doctor about being fitted for a pessary, be sure to mention whether or not you are sexually active. Your doctor will take this information into consideration and provide you with appropriate pessary choices.

Taking Care of Yourself

Because things like changes in body weight can affect how well your pessary fits, women who wear pessaries should see their doctor every six months or so for a pessary checkup. During these visits your provider will want to know if the pessary is comfortable and is helping you maintain continence. Your doctor will also physically examine you to make sure the pessary still fits properly and that the vaginal tissues look healthy.

Because a pessary is a foreign object, wearing one causes an increase in vaginal secretions. Sometimes the discharge may have a noticeable, but not foul, odor. If this becomes a problem, ask your doctor about using a prescribed odor-reducing gel.

If you have gone through menopause, declines in naturally occurring estrogen production make the vaginal tissues thin and easily injured. Be sure to tell your doctor if you feel rubbing or soreness or notice any bleeding or a foul-smelling vaginal discharge that may indicate the presence of an infection. Usually your physician can easily take care of the problems associated with menopause and thin vaginal tissues. Using an estrogen-containing vaginal cream to keep these tissues healthy is often a good long-term solution.

Although having a pessary is a safe and noninvasive way to

control stress incontinence, having one does require some upkeep and maintenance. Incorporating pessary upkeep and your regularly scheduled doctor appointments into your lifestyle can take some getting used to. However, most women find that a pessary is a welcome alternative to the daily inconvenience of coping with leaks.

Complications of Pessary Use

Fortunately, serious complications from using a pessary are few and rare. The most common problems women encounter include vaginal discharge and odor or pessary discomfort. Occasionally women may have problems urinating because the pessary oversupports the urethra. Similarly, having a bowel movement while their pessary is in place may also be difficult. More serious complications include vaginal ulceration and bleeding. It is important to see your doctor if you have vaginal bleeding when using your pessary. Ulcerations are treated by removing the pessary to allow the vaginal skin to heal. Additionally, a prescribed estrogen-containing cream will help the healing process. In extremely rare cases, women who have left their pessary in place for years without regular maintenance may need to have it surgically removed.

Remember, a pessary is a safe way to treat stress incontinence and pelvic organ prolapse. Very few women have any complications while using a pessary and pessaries can actually resolve incontinence with a single doctor visit!

Taking Care of Your Pessary

Some healthcare providers will instruct you on how to remove, clean, and reinsert your pessary. Other providers prefer that their patients come to their office every four to six weeks so they can remove, clean, and reposition the pessary for them. This is certainly a helpful service if arthritis or other conditions prevent you from having the dexterity to do this on your own.

Taking care of your pessary is not complicated. Most women can learn to insert and clean their pessary on their own. This gives you the freedom to decide when you want to wear your pessary. Some women wear their pessary during the day and remove it before going to bed or before sexual intercourse. Other women use a pessary only when they are in situations—such as exercise, gardening, or housework—that usually cause them to leak urine. Even if you opt to wear your pessary all the time, you can remove and care for your pessary without having to schedule an appointment with your doctor.

There are many benefits to learning how to remove, clean, and reinsert your pessary on your own. Regularly cleaning your pessary with warm water and soap helps keep the vaginal tissues healthy and limits the growth of odor-producing bacteria. Clinicians recommend that you do this at least once every four weeks.

Independence is another benefit. Doing your own pessary maintenance allows you to work, socialize, and travel without having to schedule frequent doctor appointments. It also feels good to know that you can take care of yourself.

Stress incontinence pessaries are generally easy to remove, clean, and insert. In fact, if you are familiar with using a contraceptive diaphragm, you already know the basic insertion and removal steps. If you never used that type of birth control—do not worry—the removal and insertion technique is easy to learn!

In either situation, it is important that you get a pessary checkup once every six months to one year. By keeping ahead of potential problems you can prolong your ability to use a pessary as a way to control stress incontinence.

MEDICATIONS

Taking certain medications can help reduce or modify bladder control problems. Some medications can be used to treat overactive bladder symptoms, while others help both the urethra and anal sphincter work more effectively to reduce incontinence symptoms. Although taking these medications can greatly improve your situation, they are not magic pills. You should continue your pelvic floor exercise regimen, scheduled urination exercises, and the diet and fluid intake management strategies that you began after reading chapter 4. Taking medications also goes hand-in-hand with physical therapy and/or wearing a pessary.

Overactive Bladder Medications

If you watch television or read magazines or newspapers you may already be familiar with some of the medications doctors prescribe to relieve overactive bladder symptoms. The advertisements make it sound so simple: you take a pill and the problem goes away.

While these medications are very helpful in reducing urgency, the side effects are sometimes bothersome enough that some women decide to stop treatment. The most common side effects— constipation and dry mouth—are related to how these drugs reduce overactive bladder symptoms.

The medications belong to a family of drugs called *anticholinergics*, which work by inhibiting the nerves that normally stimulate certain muscles to contract. Taking these medications quiets your detrusor muscle (bladder) and thus reduces urgency feelings.

Unfortunately, these medications also affect the contractile tissues located in the intestines and salivary glands. This makes it more difficult for the muscles in your intestines to dilate—or relax—and permit stool to pass. "Dry mouth" is another problem associated with taking anticholinergics. Because they inhibit saliva production, your mouth feels dry and sticky. Headaches and drowsiness are examples of other problems commonly associated with taking this class of drugs.

Before taking anticholinergic medications to relieve urgency, be sure to tell your doctor if you have sudden eye pain attacks or *narrow angle glaucoma*, heart disease, high blood pressure, intestinal problems, or an overactive thyroid. You should never take overactive bladder medications if you have narrow angle glaucoma, because doing so can cause the pressure in your eyes to increase dramatically. While it is possible to use anticholinergics if you have some of these other conditions, your provider will need to monitor your response carefully.

Although anticholinergic medications such as oxybutynin (Ditropan) and tolterodine (Detrol) are frequently prescribed to treat urgency, clinical research shows that behavioral therapy such as scheduled urination exercises is often a better approach. Not only does behavioral therapy work, it is less expensive and there are no side effects to worry about. Combining anticholinergic and behavioral therapies is another good treatment strategy.

Today, you have a variety of anticholinergic drug therapies to choose from (table 8.1). In addition to long- and short-acting preparations, some are also available in skin patches. Although it is questionable if absorbing anticholinergics through the skin is better than taking pills, patients do report fewer problems with dry mouth and constipation.

The Internet is a good way to find out more about the medications doctors prescribe to treat overactive bladder. Use either the pharmaceutical or trade names listed in table 8.1 as Internet search

Table 8.1. Medications Used to Treat Urgency

Pharmaceutical Name	Trade Name
Darifenacin	Enablex
Duloxetine (urge and stress)	Cymbalta
Oxybutynin—oral	Ditropan
Oxybutynin—skin patch	Oxytrol
Solifenacin	VESIcare
Tolterodine	Detrol
Trospium	Sanctura

prompts. When you do this, you will learn more about anticholinergic uses and side effects.

Even if you do decide to take a pharmaceutical approach to achieving continence, do not forget your pelvic floor exercises and the various behavioral and bladder management techniques you learned in chapter 4. All of these safe and cost-free strategies play an important, lifelong role in promoting pelvic floor and bladder health.

Stress Incontinence Medications

There are fewer pharmaceutical options for treating stress incontinence. Unlike overactive bladder, stress incontinence is a problem caused in part by structural or anatomical changes. This makes it difficult to find or develop medications that specifically relieve stress incontinence symptoms.

Pseudoephedrine is a medication sometimes used to relieve mild stress incontinence. Because pseudoephedrine increases the bladder neck and urethra pressures, taking it can reduce leaking.

The drug name pseudoephedrine may sound familiar to you because this substance is an active ingredient in many over-the-counter cold medications. Ephedrine, a close pharmaceutical cousin, also helps reduce stress incontinence. Ephedrine is no longer on the market because of an association with increased risk for heart attack, high blood pressure, stroke, seizures, psychosis, and death.

Using a cold medication to treat stress incontinence is an example of an *off-label use*. This is when a normally unpleasant side effect—in this case urination difficulty—can be an unexpected benefit for those trying to manage urinary incontinence. Before taking medications for off-label use, it is important to know that the Food and Drug Administration (FDA) may not have researched the safety of taking them for another purpose.

Side effects from taking pseudoephedrine can include rapid

heartbeat, anxiety and agitation, sleeplessness, increased blood pressure, headache, sweating, and difficulty breathing. You should not take pseudoephedrine to relieve cold symptoms or to treat stress incontinence without first discussing it with your doctor if you have any of the following conditions:

- High blood pressure
- Heart disease
- Kidney or liver problems
- Epilepsy or other seizure disorders
- Breathing interruptions while sleeping
- Thyroid problems
- Asthma
- Gallbladder disease
- Diabetes
- Glaucoma

Like pseudoephedrine, duloxetine is a prescription medication that has the potential to help reduce stress incontinence leaks. Because it is a medication normally prescribed to treat depression, taking duloxetine to relieve stress incontinence is another off-label drug use. Similar to pseudoephedrine, a duloxetine side effect is urination difficulty. It also has side effects such as increased blood pressure, headaches, and insomnia. Women who have high blood pressure or seizure conditions that prevent them from taking pseudoephedrine also cannot use duloxetine. Unlike pseudoephedrine, duloxetine is associated with suicidal thoughts and suicide attempts. Fortunately, this side effect rarely happens.

What about Estrogen?

Using estrogen to prevent or relieve stress incontinence is an evolving topic. Because having low estrogen blood levels is associated with tissue thinning and reduced muscle elasticity, researchers and clinicians logically thought that hormone replacement therapy (HRT) and estrogen-containing creams would prevent stress incontinence. For similar reasons they also assumed that estrogen supplements might relieve ongoing stress incontinence symptoms. Research shows these assumptions are not true.

Although estrogen is no longer a stress incontinence remedy, creams containing estrogen do increase the ability of postmenopausal women to insert, wear, and remove a pessary successfully. In addition to providing lubrication, these creams make the vaginal tissues less susceptible to tearing and decrease problems with pain, bleeding, and the development of skin ulcers. Therefore, many doctors prescribe estrogen creams to help patients successfully wear a pessary.

MONITERING YOUR PROGRESS

By now you have learned about and maybe even tried several incontinence treatment strategies. Some of these strategies are things you did at home and others you did with the help of your healthcare provider. Consider completing Worksheet 8A at the end of the chapter to document the progress you have made with bladder control. Doing so will help you to set goals and monitor your progress thus far as well as identify management strategies that you still might like to try. Remember that regaining bladder control often takes a combination of therapies—there really are no magic pills!

DO I NEED ANOTHER SOLUTION?

"I have tried everything. Doing pelvic floor exercises, making diet changes, diligently following my scheduled urinations, trying to use a pessary, and even going to physical therapy haven't worked. I still leak. What other options do I have?"

Unfortunately, some women find that even after all this effort, and hopefully some degree of improvement, they are not able to manage their stress incontinence satisfactorily. For these women surgery may be the next option.

The decision to undergo a surgical procedure is not always an easy one. Stress incontinence surgeries range from outpatient procedures such as bulking agent injections to rigorous pelvic floor reconstructions. No surgical procedure comes with a guarantee.

Knowing this caused one patient to say, "I don't want to risk what I have for something I might have." For her, the uncertainty of a successful surgical outcome made her think more favorably about pelvic floor exercises and pessaries.

However, for other women, bladder stress tests may reveal that surgery is their only chance to regain continence. For them, making the decision to undergo surgery gives them hope.

In the next chapter, you will learn about the procedures surgeons use to reduce stress incontinence. You will also learn how to find a qualified surgeon and to prepare yourself for surgery and recovery.

WORKSHEETS

Worksheet 8A: Evaluating My Progress

You have learned about and maybe even tried several incontinence treatment strategies. Some of these strategies are things you did at home and others you did with the help of your healthcare provider.

Since the next chapter discusses surgical solutions, this is a good time to evaluate the progress you have made so far.

At-Home Strategies

Pelvic Floor Exercises

1. I do _____ pelvic floor exercise repeat sets each day. (give number)

2. I have been doing daily pelvic floor exercises for: (check one)
___ days
___ weeks
___ months

3. Pelvic floor exercise helps me successfully control urgency. (circle one) Yes / No

4. Since beginning daily pelvic floor exercises, urine leaking and accidents are: (check one)
___ fewer
___ increased
___ no change

5. Since beginning pelvic floor exercises I feel that I have: (check one)

___ better bladder control
___ less bladder control
___ no change

Scheduled Urination Exercises

1. Since completing my scheduled urination exercises I go to the bathroom to urinate: (circle one) (less often than before), (more often than before).

2. Since completing my scheduled urination exercises, urgency and bladder control is: (check one)
    ___ improved
    ___ worse
    ___ no change

I know this because I can now wait _____ hours before having to go to the bathroom.

Healthcare-Provided Strategies

Physical Therapy

1. I have tried biofeedback as a way to improve how I do pelvic floor exercises: (circle one) Yes / No

2. Biofeedback has made it easier for me to identify and exercise my pelvic floor muscles: (circle one) Yes / No

3. Now that I have completed my biofeedback therapy my ability to control my bladder has: (check one)
    ___ improved
    ___ worse
    ___ no change

I know this because: _____

_____

4. I have tried electrostimulation as a way to reduce urge: (circle one) Yes / No

5. Now that I have completed my electrostimulation therapy, problems with overactive bladder urgency have: (check one)
___ improved
___ worse
___ no change

I know this because: _____

_____

Pessary

1. I am using a pessary to relieve stress incontinence: (circle one) Yes / No

2. Since wearing a pessary I have bladder accidents: (check one)
___ less often than before
___ more often than before
___ unchanged

3. Since wearing a pessary the amount of urine I leak is: (check one)
___ less
___ more
___ the same

4. I believe a pessary has improved my independence and quality of life: (circle one) Yes / No

I know this because: _____

_____

Medication

1. I am taking medication to help control overactive bladder urgency: (circle one) Yes / No

2. I have improvement: (circle one) Yes / No

I have the following improvements: _____

_____

I have side effects: (circle one) Yes / No

I have the following side effects: _____

_____

Overall, I find the side effects manageable and worth the outcome: (circle one) Yes / No

3. I am taking medication to help control stress incontinence: (circle one) Yes / No

I have the following improvements: _____

_____

I have the following side effects: _____

_____

Overall, I find the side effects manageable and worth the outcome: (circle one) Yes / No

4. Taking medication has improved my overactive bladder condition: (circle one) Yes / No / NA

I know this because: _____

_____

5. Taking medication has made stress incontinence manageable: (circle one) Yes / No

I know this because: _____

_____

Questions for Self-evaluation and Reflection

1. Is my bladder control better than before?

_____

_____

2. Is it good enough?

_____

_____

3. Are my bladder control problems manageable?

_____

_____

4. Does incontinence still affect my ability to socialize, be intimate with my partner, or do my job?

_____

_____

5. Do I want to consider a surgical treatment at this time?

_____

_____

6. What do I expect to achieve from having surgery?

_____

_____

7. What is a "good enough" result?

_____

_____

FREQUENTLY ASKED QUESTIONS

1. How long will it take for treatments to work?

As with any other lifestyle or health adjustment you might make, your urinary incontinence treatment results will depend on many factors. One important factor may be your level of motivation! With these treatments, active patient participation is vital. Other factors include the severity of your condition, your overall health, and your access to the necessary medical treatments.

2. It seems like every time I go to the doctor I get new or different information. What is happening?

Doctors modify and change their treatment strategies in response to new information. The use of long-term hormone replacement therapy (HRT) is a good example that demonstrates how medical research can change patient treatment. Once thought to provide health protection for women, studies now show that taking hormone replacement therapy after menopause slightly increases a woman's risk for a heart attack, breast cancer, and stress incontinence. While no longer considered an appropriate incontinence treatment, hormone replacement therapy does reduce hot flashes and excessive bleeding. Short-term hormone replacement therapy is still an important menopause management strategy. However, like all medications it has risks and benefits.

3. Do health insurance policies cover treatments such as biofeedback and electrostimulation?

Typically, health insurance policies cover these treatments. However, it is always good to check what your policy covers beforehand.

4. Are there any side effects associated with pelvic floor exercises, biofeedback, and electrostimulation treatments?

No, all are safe treatments without known adverse side effects.

5. Can the pessary get lost inside of me?

No. Because the vagina is like a pocket, the pessary can get no further than the back of the vagina. However, a pessary that is too small can fall out of your vagina. If this should happen—clean it with soap and water and put it back. You should also make an appointment to get a better-fitting pessary.

6. How much does a pessary cost?

The catalogue prices for most pessaries are between $50 and $100.

7. How long does a pessary last before I need a new one?

How long a pessary lasts depends on many factors that include changes in body weight and in your pelvic floor. Assuming everything is stable, a pessary should last for many years.

8. Should I wear my pessary at night?

Wearing a pessary at night is your decision.

9. How is an incontinence pessary different from the diaphragm I once used to prevent pregnancy?

An incontinence pessary does not prevent pregnancy because sperm can travel through it. A diaphragm is a flexible dome-shaped cup made of rubber or plastic that fits over the uterine cervix. To prevent pregnancy you fill the diaphragm cup with a spermicidal cream.

10. What medications can I use to reduce stress incontinence if I have epilepsy, high blood pressure, or any of the other listed conditions?

You will need to discuss your situation with your doctor or other healthcare provider. Your doctor will carefully evaluate how any stress incontinence medications might interact with or lead to dangerous side effects in association with your current medications.

11. Why does being diabetic make bladder control more difficult?

This is a complicated question to answer, because not everyone has the same kind of diabetes or the same severity of disease. However, in general diabetic women make more urine when their sugars are not well controlled, which can lead to more accidents. Women with diabetes also have slow damage to the nerves and muscles of the entire body—including the bladder—which can lead to difficulty emptying the bladder, decreased sensation in the bladder, and increased overactivity.

12. How can I find out about participating in a clinical incontinence drug trial study?

You can often find advertisements in your local paper when medical centers and large medical practices are looking for people willing to take part in new drug studies. Participating in clinical trial studies helps the Food and Drug Administration evaluate the effectiveness and safety of new medications.

In addition to newspapers, the Internet is another resource for finding local clinical trial sites. Using word prompts such as "incontinence" and "clinical trials" is a good way to find urinary incontinence drug study locations throughout the United States. You can make your search even more efficient by also adding your state or city to your query.

Not everyone can participate in an incontinence clinical trial study. Criteria such as gender, age, medical history, and willingness to undergo medical tests are common selective factors. Because these are controlled studies, participants do not know if they are in the group that actually receives the new medication. This is another factor you need to take into consideration before you decide to volunteer.

13. Can I take urgency medications to help me manage stress incontinence?

Usually this is not helpful. But doctors have noticed that sometimes taking medications meant for urge incontinence can help reduce stress incontinence. Taking these medications for this purpose is an off-label use and should be discussed thoroughly with your healthcare professional.

14. If I have trouble emptying my bladder can I use anticholinergic medications to help reduce my urgency symptoms?

It depends. To find out, your healthcare provider may do a postvoid residual test (see chapter 6) to check how well your bladder empties as well as to monitor how well your bladder empties after you start taking the anticholinergic.

CHAPTER 9

WHEN SURGERY IS YOUR BEST OPTION

*"There comes a point when you acquiesce.
All the worrying stops when you walk
through the hospital door. "*
Barbara—A medical social worker and incontinence patient

ANOTHER TURNING POINT

❝**I** am just plain tired of all this! My pessary isn't working as well as it used to. Now, when I cough or sneeze I leak urine. I hate having to deal with pads but—if I don't use them—I constantly worry about wet spots. Maybe I should retire and just stay home."

Margaret, a successful real estate agent and grandmother, has come to the point where she needs to make an important decision. Although she enjoys helping clients find and purchase a new home, her bladder control problems make concentrating on work difficult. Managing stress incontinence also puts a dent in her relationship with her grandchildren. Once an avid hiker and cyclist, she has always envisioned taking her grandchildren on some memorable adventures. Now, even having that pleasure seems unlikely.

Talking to some longtime friends about their stress incontinence surgeries helped make Margaret feel less apprehensive about taking a similar route. One friend had just returned to work after having some kind of day-surgery procedure little more than a week ago. Another friend, whose surgery required staying a few days in the hospital, exclaimed that "she wished she had done this for herself years ago."

Their enthusiasm and earnest desire to give helpful advice was both surprising and encouraging. "It is such a relief to know that other options are available," Margaret thought to herself.

WHEN IS SURGERY MY BEST OPTION?

It is worthwhile to consider surgery when nonsurgical treatments are not giving you the desired level of control or when incontinence continues to have a negative impact on your life. Some women choose surgery as their first option. Without question, the decision to have surgery—or not to—is both a personal and subjective matter. What is important to remember is that you have many options for bladder control treatment.

Making the decision to undergo a surgical procedure is never easy. Many women who put off even considering a surgical solution say afterward that they wished they had decided to have the surgery much sooner. For some patients, because of the nature of their bladder control problems, having surgery is their only hope for regaining continence. For others, dietary changes, weight loss, behavioral modification, pessaries, or overactive bladder did not produce an acceptable level of bladder control. In either case, your decision to undergo surgery is not an admission of inability to follow your doctor's recommendations or personal weakness or failure.

Although the choice is always yours to make, your doctor and undoubtedly your friends and family will have something to say about it. Your doctor can provide information, advice, and suggest that you explore various options. Look to your friends and family for encouragement and support.

It is important to remember that surgery is a stress incontinence treatment option. Overactive bladder cannot be treated with surgery. However, one exception to this rule is a surgical procedure called *neuromodulation*. This is when a surgically implanted electric pulse generator, similar to ones used to control back pain, is used to relieve otherwise resistant overactive bladder symptoms. Keep in mind that the success or failure of someone else's surgical repair should not overly influence your thoughts. Every situation is different because of individual differences in anatomy and function, thereby making every incontinence surgery a "custom job."

AN OVERVIEW OF SURGICAL TREATMENTS FOR INCONTINENCE

Surgical procedures to help women cope with stress incontinence have been available for nearly one hundred years. In 1913, Dr. Howard A. Kelly devised a method using stitched-in pleats to narrow the bladder neck to treat stress incontinence. Later, surgeons devised other techniques to support and elevate the bladder neck and urethra. Many of the nearly one hundred different incontinence procedures that are available to you today are refinements of these earlier surgical strategies.

Early-twentieth-century surgeries involved large abdominal incisions. Today, improved surgical tools and techniques allow surgeons to enter the *pelvic cavity* through the vagina or the abdomen. Using a *laparoscope* to see into the pelvic cavity enables surgeons to perform many incontinence surgeries through several small abdominal and vaginal incisions.

The bottom line is, no matter what procedures your surgeon uses, the goal is to improve urinary continence. They need to accomplish this with the smallest risk for complications and without inadvertently creating new bladder control problems.

SURGEONS AND INCONTINENCE SURGERY

It is important that your clinician use the best methods available for your incontinence treatment. These are not necessarily the newest therapies, but they are ones that many surgeons can successfully perform; they have low complication rates; and their long-term effectiveness has been established. Talk to your doctor about these crucial aspects of your treatment. It is also very important that you trust your surgeon and feel comfortable working with his or her office and staff. Use Worksheet 9A (see p. 262) to help organize your thoughts on this important topic. Doing so can help you decide if this surgical practice, in terms of such things as location, patient services, and other patient management procedures, meets your needs.

Like clinicians who train to become pediatricians, cardiologists, or family practitioners, surgeons also have specialties. Knowing what types of surgical specialists treat female incontinence will help you find a surgeon who can provide the best treatment tailored to meet your specific needs.

General surgeons usually perform abdominal-area surgeries such as appendectomies, hernias, and assorted trauma repairs. Although some general surgeons perform female reproductive tract surgeries, most do not. If you are seeing a general surgeon, you need to find out if that person frequently performs incontinence surgeries.

Gynecologists do everything from providing birth control information, treating sexually transmitted diseases, and delivering babies to performing hysterectomies and other surgeries involving the female reproductive organs. Many gynecologists also treat incontinence and pelvic floor disorders.

Urogynecology is a gynecological subspecialty that requires three more years of training after completing a four-year gynecology residency. Urogynecologists specialize in caring for women who have urinary or anal incontinence, urinary frequency problems, pelvic organ prolapse, and pelvic pain.

Many urologists treat female urinary incontinence. These doctors may also treat male infertility, and treat men and women for kidney disease, urinary tract cancers, and urinary tract stones. Female urology is a urology specialty that requires one to two years of additional training after a five-year residency. If possible, look for a urologist who also specializes in treating female urinary tract problems.

You have many choices. It is therefore important to select a clinician or a medical group with a demonstrated interest in treating female incontinence and a proven track record in surgical and non-surgical treatments.

Talking to your primary care doctor can be a good place to start. Other sources of information include medical center gynecology or urology departments in large medical centers and referrals from friends and family members. As you can see, learning as much as possible about your options will help you to make good medical care decisions. Refer to chapters 4, 5, and 6 for more help on this subject.

GETTING READY FOR SURGERY

Preparing for surgery is both a physical and a mental process. Although most providers do not discuss these aspects of surgical readiness, it is beneficial if you enter surgery as physically healthy as possible. You also need to get emotionally ready to undergo what is by all standards a scary experience. And then there are practical issues—getting food in the house, arranging for your household and work responsibilities, and finally completing all the things you must do just before going to the hospital.

It Is a Process

Getting ready for surgery is a slow and subtle process. Sometimes it helps to talk to understanding and supportive friends and family. Your provider may recommend a local support group or a practice-based patient education class to help you learn more about incontinence surgeries. However, be selective and try to seek information from people who you feel are reliable sources of information. We all know that too much advice and too many "gory" stories get in the way of clear thinking.

There are many things that you can do to decrease feelings of presurgical apprehension. Plan what you'll do after surgery—lunch with friends, reading good books, and enjoying movies or other quiet and pleasurable activities. It is also helpful to think of all the women who have already benefited from incontinence surgeries. Like you, these women made the decision to undergo a surgical treatment. In time, the moments of fear and worry will lessen and your focus will shift from the "day of surgery" to looking forward to "days of improved continence."

Practical Readiness

Work, home, and family—women tend to prepare for "down time." Do not let presurgical preparations become an overwhelming undertaking. Ask your surgeon about your expected recovery time and postsurgical physical limitations. Doing this will help you make realistic plans.

Accept the help of others. Identify important tasks and ignore things that really do not matter. Although easier said than done, this approach will help your recovery and healing process. Inform your colleagues and coworkers of your upcoming absence. You or your supervisor can delegate duties and adjust work schedules to accommodate workplace needs. If possible, try to avoid having big presurgical or postrecovery deadlines to deal with.

At home, tell family members what they can do to be helpful. Give them a "to do" list and a list of useful or important phone numbers. However, be considerate of their time and understanding of their emotional strain. Try to remember that a "tidy and orderly" house may not be one of the most important things to worry about at this time.

It can be helpful to hire a cleaning service or pay a driver to run errands. Buy or make food ahead of time to keep in the freezer. Collect phone numbers of restaurants with good take-out services. Use Worksheet 9B (on p. 266) to help organize your presurgical preparations. Doing so will help make your hospitalization and recovery easier for yourself, your family, and your work colleagues.

READY AND WAITING

Before your surgery, you will receive presurgical instructions from your doctor's nurse or from the hospital patient education nurse. This is a good time to ask questions and to remind your healthcare provider about special needs and concerns. It is very important that they know about every prescription, over-the-counter, and herbal medication that you take.

You should also tell your doctor of any other medical conditions you have, such as high blood pressure, diabetes, or epilepsy. Even if you have told them before, a reminder will not hurt. Your doctor needs this information to give you the best possible care before, during, and after your surgery. In addition, you may have last-minute questions for your doctor. Worksheet 9C (p. 270) provides a list of questions that will reveal gaps in your understanding and gives you the opportunity to ask any remaining questions or review instructions with your doctor and other clinical staff.

You will be told not to eat or drink anything other than water for at least six hours before your procedure. Going into surgery on an empty stomach makes it less likely that you will vomit while under anesthesia. Vomiting is a potentially dangerous situation, because you could inhale stomach contents into your lungs.

Depending on the surgical procedure and your doctor's personal preference, you may need to give yourself an *enema* the evening before going to the hospital. When under general anesthesia, your bowels are on "automatic pilot" and you cannot control defecation. An unexpected bowel movement, aside from distracting the surgeon, can dirty the surgical area and increase your risk for infection.

Try to relax the day before your surgery. This is a good time to do pleasurable activities. Spend the evening with friends. Go to a movie or a concert. Play cards, watch television, or work on a favorite home project.

Now the day has come and you are ready to have your surgery. It is time to give yourself to trusted hands. A friend or a family member takes you to the hospital. You arrive, with few personal effects, and go to a designated waiting area. A nurse calls your name and the big day begins.

After you put on a surgical gown, head covering, and booties, a nurse escorts you and a family member into the surgery preparation area. Lying on a *gurney* and covered by a light blanket, you wait. Soon a nurse comes by to ask questions and to take and record your temperature, pulse, and blood pressure. Your surgeon, on the way to the operating room, stops by to say hello.

The anesthesiologist is your next visitor. More questions. The anesthesiologist wants to know about the last time you ate, your drinking and smoking habits, and if you have loose teeth or removable dental work. This same doctor also asks you about your overall health, the medications you take, the location of old injuries, and your reactions to certain drugs. Your anesthesiologist uses this information to decide on the type and amount of anesthesia, and the best way to position you on the surgical table. This information also helps the anesthesiologist to anticipate if the placement of an *endotracheal tube* might cause you to lose and then swallow loose teeth.

To prevent the possibility of damage to dental work, patients are asked to take out their dentures and removable bridges.

After signing procedural consent papers, the anesthesiologist gives you a light sedative. While you relax, the nurses prepare the surgical suite for your arrival and the surgeons scrub their hands and arms to prepare themselves for the work ahead.

AN OVERVIEW OF
INCONTINENCE SURGICAL PROCEDURES

There are many surgical incontinence treatment approaches. Some, such as bulking agents and *mid-urethral* sling procedures, are minimally invasive. Others, many of which are *retropubic* procedures, are major surgeries.

Which procedure, or combinations of procedures, your doctor uses depends on the underlying causes of your incontinence. And as you will see later, having pelvic organ prolapse, a condition that often accompanies urinary incontinence, may indicate the necessity of more invasive and extensive surgical strategies.

While you may not be invited into the decision-making process regarding the specific surgical procedures you need, your surgeon should explain the "hows" and "whys" of your upcoming surgery. Ask questions so that your surgeon can clarify and explain more fully those aspects of the surgery that you do not understand. Sometimes it is helpful to bring a friend or family member to take notes and to act as a second set of ears.

Making Your Urethra Tighter: Bulking Agents

Bulking agents are the best surgical option for women who have a well-supported bladder and an immobile urethra to get stress incontinence relief. While bulking agents are a treatment option for women who have a mobile urethra, other surgeries have higher success rates. Currently there are two types of bulking agents—collagen (a skin and bone protein from cows) and carbon-coated beads. Research is underway to develop additional types of injectable bulking agents.

Perhaps you have already heard of the collagen injections that dermatologists and cosmetic surgeons use to remove wrinkles. This time, instead of filling out your "character lines" your doctor is "filling in" the upper part of your urethra. This procedure helps control your urine flow by narrowing the opening of the bladder neck (fig. 9.1), the tube that connects your bladder to the urethra (figs. 9.2a and 9.2b).

While usually a hospital procedure, some doctors provide bulking agent injections in their office. To prevent pain, your doctor, or an anesthesiologist, will give you a local anesthetic and/or intravenous sedation. After you have reached an appropriate

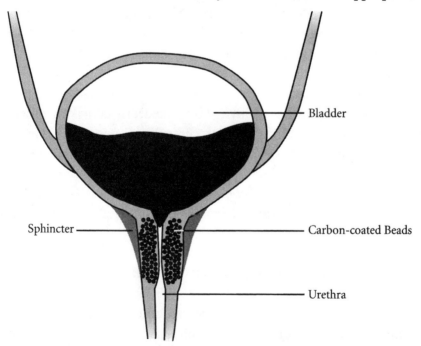

Fig. 9.1. Bulking agent injections help control your urine flow by narrowing the opening of the bladder neck.

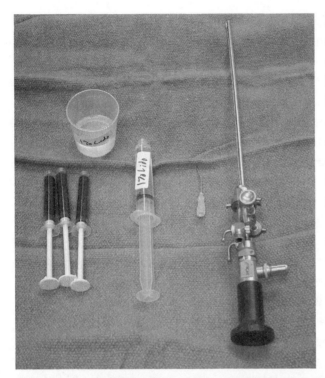

Fig. 9.2a. Getting ready for carbon-coated bead injections. From left to right: syringes containing carbon-coated beads, saline, and on the right, a cysto-scope that allows the doctor to see inside the bladder and the bladder neck.

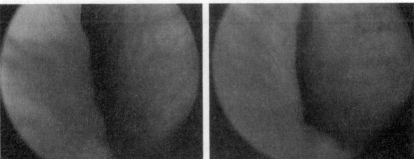

Fig. 9.2b. These photos—taken through a cystoscope—show (*left*) a large bladder neck opening and (*right*) after carbon-coated bead injection, a smaller bladder neck opening.

level of sedation, your doctor will insert a cystoscope, through the urethra and into the bladder. The cystoscope is used to visually check for bladder abnormalities that might be contributing to your incontinence. To perform the injection, the cystoscope is pulled back to just below the bladder neck. The injection is made into the surrounding urethral tissues on either side of the bladder neck. The bubble of injected material produces a localized swelling that helps you to have a more controlled urine flow.

Although collagen and carbon-coated bead injections are relatively simple procedures, you still need some preoperative preparation. A few days before your surgery you will need to have a urine test to make sure you do not have a urinary tract infection. Be sure to tell your doctor if you experience pain when urinating or are urinating with greater frequency. If you have a urinary tract infection, you will have to wait until the infection has cleared up before you can undergo surgery.

Collagen injections require a little more preoperative preparation than carbon-coated bead injections. Because cow collagen is not identical to human collagen, some women are sensitive to it. About four weeks before your injections, your doctor needs to find out if you are sensitive or allergic to this protein.

Although most women can safely use this product, the collagen skin test identifies those who are allergic to this natural protein. For this test, a healthcare provider will ask if you are allergic to beef or cow's milk, to surgical materials such as sutures, or have a history of rheumatoid arthritis or systemic lupus. The office nurse will perform a simple test, similar to an allergy skin test, to make sure that collagen is a safe material for you. To do this, the nurse injects a small under-the-skin collagen bubble on the palm-side of your forearm.

You will need to observe the injection site carefully and frequently for redness, firmness, tenderness, swelling, and itching for the first three days after the injection and at least once a day for the next twenty-eight days. The nurse may also provide a questionnaire to help you keep track of your observations. Negative test results means that you are less likely to have an allergic reaction to these injections. This kind of testing is not necessary if you are going to receive carbon-coated bead injections.

After your bulking agent injections, a nurse will take you to a recovery area. You will need to wait for the anesthesia to wear off and be able to urinate before going home. If you cannot urinate, a nurse will insert a urinary catheter or show you how to *self-catheterize*. You cannot go home until you are able to urinate normally or can show that you can self-catheterize.

During the first twenty-four hours after receiving bulking agent injections, you may experience some changes in your urination pattern. Localized swelling, the way our body responds to surgery, may cause temporary urination difficulties and feelings of urgency. You may also experience injection-site soreness and observe slight urethral bleeding and small amounts of blood in your urine. Call your doctor if these symptoms persist for more than a few days.

After carbon-bead injections, some women notice black specks in the toilet or on a pad. This leakage of excess carbon beads is normal for the first few days after surgery.

Some postsurgical signs and symptoms are indicators of potentially serious problems. Immediately tell your doctor if you have cloudy or foul-smelling urine or if you have a fever above 101 degrees Fahrenheit. These are signs of a urinary tract infection. You need to take antibiotics to treat the infection.

Another area for concern is allergic reactions to collagen injections. This is a rare occurrence, but you should call your doctor if you experience:

- Joint pain or joint swelling
- Skin rash or skin thickening
- Muscle aches, fever, weakness, or fatigue

Supporting Your Urethra: Mid-urethral Slings

Mid-urethral slings are a relatively new way to treat stress incontinence. By repositioning and supporting the urethra, mid-urethral slings increase urethral pressure and prevent bladder leakage (fig. 9.3).

Mid-urethral slings are an appropriate treatment for women who have stress incontinence resulting from having a mobile and/or weakened urethra. Having a mobile urethra makes it harder to counteract increased bladder pressure. Some women, in addition to having a mobile urethra, may also have a weakened or low-pressure urethra. As you may recall from chapter 3, having either of these problems will make bladder control difficult because the urethra cannot effectively prevent urine from leaking. Mid-urethral slings can be used when other medical management methods have failed to provide sufficient relief. You can undergo this procedure either by itself or in combination with other pelvic floor repairs.

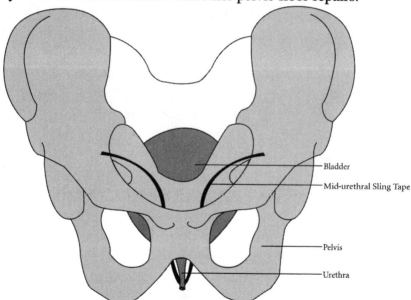

Fig. 9.3. This is what a supportive transvaginal tape looks like placed inside your body.

Although more invasive than bulking agent injections, mid-ure-thral slings involve weaving a supportive ribbon under the midportion of the urethra. Depending on the specific type of mid-urethral sling procedure, support materials range from fabricated *polypropylene* meshlike ribbons to fibrous tissue pieces taken from your own body or other animal sources.

The *transvaginal tape sling*, or TVT, is the most commonly performed and best-studied mid-urethral sling. For this procedure, the surgeon makes two very small incisions into your lower abdomen just above your pubic bone. A third incision in the vagina provides access to the urethra.

Using a pair of guiding needles, the surgeon threads a ribbon of polypropylene mesh fabric through the vaginal incision (fig. 9.4). The surgeon positions the ribbon-carrying needles so the ribbon cradles the urethra as the needles emerge through the abdominal incisions. Supporting the middle section of the urethra helps the urethra to stay closed when you cough or sneeze, and prevents involuntary urine loss.

Transobturator tape is another mid-urethral sling procedure. The main difference between the two methods is the location of the entry-point incisions. For a transobturator tape sling, the surgeon makes incisions just below your pubic bone and threads the sling material through naturally occurring holes located on both sides of your *pelvis*.

Unlike other more invasive surgical procedures, the surgeon does not stitch or tack the support material to structurally stable tissues or bone. In this case, the rough-textured mesh provides support by increasing friction, which decreases organ movement. Over time, your body deposits collagen in and around the polypropylene mesh. This helps to permanently position the polypropylene support ribbon within the surrounding tissues.

In addition to transvaginal and transobturator tape slings there are other mid-urethral sling procedures and products. While many use meshlike fabric ribbons to position and support the urethra,

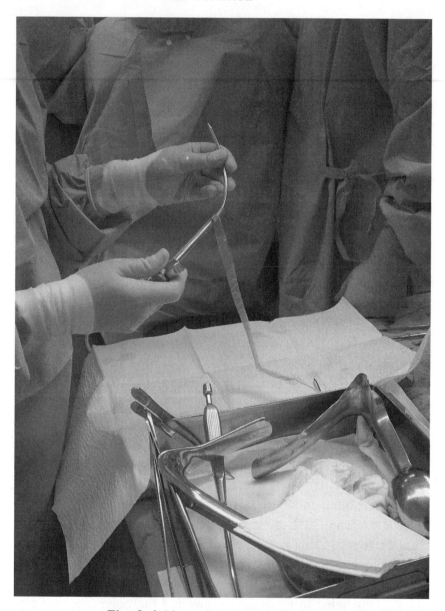

Fig. 9.4. Here the surgeon is threading the TVT-guiding needle with the polypropylene ribbon attached. The ribbon will help reposition and support the urethra.

there are subtle variations in how the surgeon inserts them. The newer mid-urethral sling products are designed to reduce complications such as bladder perforations by the guiding needles. These products have not been used long enough for researchers to support or refute the benefits of using them.

However, there is enough clinical evidence to support the effectiveness and safety of the original transvaginal tape procedure. Clinical data show that even seven years after their surgery, up to 85 percent of women receiving a transvaginal tape procedure report a "cure" or significant improvement of their stress incontinence symptoms.

In general, mid-urethral techniques offer many advantages. Unlike more invasive incontinence surgeries, the mid-urethral sling is an outpatient procedure that takes less than an hour to perform.

Although you can undergo a mid-urethral sling procedure with general anesthesia, using local anesthesia and light sedation allows you to respond to your surgeon's directions and to cough when asked. This helps the surgeon to place the support tape where you will get the most benefit.

Mid-urethral slings are not an appropriate remedy for all women. Doctors do not recommend this type of procedure for young women who are still growing, women who are or who plan to become pregnant, or for women who must take blood-thinning drugs such as heparin or warfarin (Coumadin).

Minimal preparation is needed for a mid-urethral sling procedure. Your provider should test your urine for bacteria to make sure you do not have a urinary tract infection, and if appropriate, give you a pregnancy test. Urinary tract infections must be treated and fully cleared before you can undergo this procedure.

After your mid-urethral sling has been inserted, a nurse will take you to the office or hospital recovery area. You will need to wait for the anesthesia to wear off and be able to urinate before going home. If you cannot urinate, a nurse will use a catheter to empty your bladder. The nurse may also show you how to insert and use a catheter so you can self-catheterize at home.

After you get home, you should rest and take pain medication as needed. Although full recovery usually takes about two weeks, you can do most of your daily activities after one week. However, you should follow your doctor's directions about lifting and sexual intercourse. Medical leave, depending on your work environment, ranges from one to four weeks.

Like any other surgery, there are risks associated with having this relatively noninvasive procedure. Although occurring infrequently, some surgical and postsurgical complications include bladder perforation; erosion of the mesh into the vagina, urethra, or bladder; urine retention; overactive bladder symptoms; bleeding; and infections. Your doctor may be able to correct urine retention problems by adjusting the tape's tension or cutting the tape. Usually cutting the tape resolves the urine retention problem without reversing the surgery. But sometimes cutting the tape does allow incontinence to return. You should report bleeding, abdominal pain, foul-smelling urine, urinary urgency, and fever to your doctor.

Retropubic Procedures

Bulking agents and mid-urethral slings are not the answer for all women. Some require more extensive repairs. Others, even when given the option of receiving a less invasive mid-urethral sling, opt for a procedure that surgeons have used for many years. Other women feel uneasy about having polypropylene and other materials permanently implanted in their lower abdomen.

Treating stress incontinence with a retropubic procedure means that the surgeon enters the pelvic cavity through the abdomen. To limit urethral movement and to establish a better angle between the bladder and the bladder neck, the surgeon uses the tissues on both sides of the urethra to lift the urethra into a better position. Several well-placed stitches between this tissue and the *ligaments* above it provide a hammock of support.

Some retropubic techniques require large abdominal incisions and others use laparoscopes inserted through tiny abdominal incisions. Some surgeons find that performing the operation through an abdominal incision gives better long-term results. Other surgeons have good results using laparoscopic procedures. While there are no certain answers, your surgeon should be able to explain why they have chosen a particular surgical technique for you.

Patients who have severe stress incontinence may require other stabilization procedures to achieve bladder control. To help these patients, the surgeon may use a traditional sub-urethral sling method to create bladder support. This operation is similar to the mid-urethral sling procedures except that the surgeon places the support material at the bladder neck rather than at the mid-urethra.

Based on your personal combination of incontinence problems, the surgeon will decide which type of support material will work best to suit your unique needs. Support materials can include fibrous tissue called *fascia*, which can be removed from your abdomen, leg, or is specially preserved cadaver tissue, or synthetic fibrous meshes. The support material is then placed at the bladder neck to support the urethra (fig. 9.6).

Although you may not have a large abdominal scar to remind you, these procedures are "major surgery." Patients may receive a spinal block or general anesthesia to control pain. It usually takes the surgeon between one and two hours to complete these procedures.

Sacral Neuromodulation for Urgency

Neuromodulation can relieve urgency when methods such as scheduled urination exercises, dietary changes, and medications fail to help. Neuromodulation, like the electrostimulation therapy described in chapter 8, uses electricity to reduce urgency. Similar to receiving a heart pacemaker, neuromodulation requires the surgical placement of a stopwatch-sized implantable pulse generator under the skin to stimulate the sacral nerve with small and repetitive electric impulses that quiet the nerve and inhibit urgency. These nerves

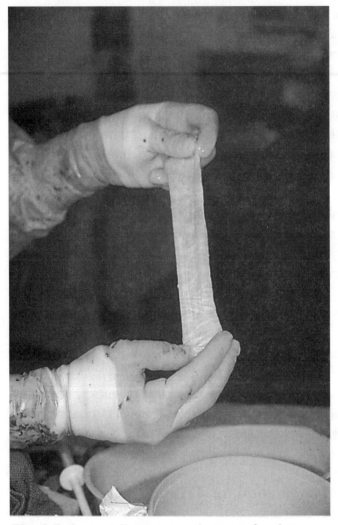

Fig. 9.5. A specially preserved piece of cadaver fascia is sometimes used to provide bladder support with a traditional sub-urethral sling procedure.

are located in the lower part of your back, just above your tailbone, and are an important part of the brain-bladder communication system discussed in chapters 2 and 3.

You can undergo sacral neuromodulation on a trial basis. If you opt for this treatment, your surgeon inserts a thin wire near the sacral nerve and then connects it to an external current generator. Getting outfitted for a sacral neuromodulation trial is usually an office procedure that takes about thirty minutes to complete. Similar to using electrical stimulation to control back pain, you wear the sacral nerve stimulator on a belt. During this trial period be sure to keep a bladder diary. Your daily record of the number of times you go to the bathroom to urinate, or have leaks or accidents is a good indicator of whether or not sacral neuromodulation will help you. Comparing the results of your neuromodulation bladder diary to your original bladder diary is an especially helpful evaluation tool. Usually a one-week trial is long enough to find out if this method will work for you.

If the external generator does reduce urgency, leaking, or accidents, then you may want to consider having an implantable pulse generator placed in your upper buttock, which makes it both inconspicuous and compatible with most types of clothing. After making a small incision, the surgeon slides the intermittent pulse generator under a skin flap and threads a wire under your skin from the generator to the sacral nerve.

Installing an intermittent pulse generator is an outpatient procedure usually requiring only local anesthesia. However, just like preparing for any surgery, your healthcare provider will give you instructions to follow prior to and after the procedure.

Using an implantable pulse generator does not interfere with sitting or sleeping positions. It also does not prevent you from participating in sports or other physical activities. You or your doctor can fine-tune pulse generation to meet your exact needs. This therapy is reversible, and the implant is removable.

INCONTINENCE WITH PELVIC ORGAN PROLAPSE SURGERY

As you learned in chapter 7, pelvic organ prolapse often accompanies stress incontinence. When this is the case, your surgery will be more extensive. In addition to stabilizing and repositioning the urethra, the surgeon will attempt to anchor sagging tissues to stable bones and ligaments. This is a little bit like reattaching sagging window drapery to a sturdy curtain rod.

Many times, based on your symptoms, physical exam, and medical imaging studies, the surgeon will know exactly which areas need repair. Other times, your surgeon will discover additional prolapsed areas during the operation that may or may not need repair.

Unfortunately for some women, surgical treatment for pelvic organ prolapse are an ongoing project. While the first surgery is performed to repair the obvious problems, some women may need additional surgery later as other pelvic organs begin to sag.

Prolapse repairs increase the time you are in the operating room. Instead of a thirty- to sixty-minute operation, this surgery may take two to four hours to complete. Your hospital stay and at-home recovery will also be longer.

HYSTERECTOMIES

A hysterectomy is not an incontinence or prolapse repair procedure. Removing your uterus is unlikely to improve bladder control and may in fact increase the risk of complications. If you have problems with excessive uterine bleeding, fibroids, or other noncancerous uterine growths, or pain, it may be appropriate to have a hysterectomy at this time.

However, if you require extensive prolapse surgery, then having a hysterectomy at this time may be suggested. Research shows that removing the uterus under these conditions often produces a better surgical repair for pelvic organ prolapse. The uterus, although it may have moved downward, does not cause pelvic organ pro-lapse—it rides the prolapse out of the vaginal opening. Simply removing the prolapsed or "fallen" uterus does not reattach the sag-ging vagina to its supports.

Be sure to talk to your surgeon about the necessity of having a hysterectomy whether or not you have a strong opinion about this aspect of your incontinence and prolapse surgery. Sources of infor-mation and names of local specialists who are comfortable per-forming incontinence repairs without a hysterectomy include the Society of Gynecological Surgeons, the American Urogynecolog-ical Association, and the American Urological Society.

THE BIG DAY

Operating suites are busy places. Between scheduled surgeries, the orderlies and surgical technologists disinfect the room, remove the trash and medical waste, and take used surgical gowns and soiled linens to the hospital laundry.

Now the operating room is clean and other clinical staff gets ready for your arrival. A gowned, masked, and gloved surgical technologist collects and arranges the instruments and supplies your surgeon needs to perform your surgery. With everything arranged on draped tables, it looks like the surgical technologist is preparing the flatware for a well-orchestrated dinner party.

The scrub nurse works closely with other team members and makes sure that there are enough supplies and medications on hand. The scrub nurse is also responsible for the paperwork that will become part of your medical record. During the surgery, this nurse answers the phone, replenishes supplies, and keeps a tally of the used needles and gauzes.

There are many other nurses and surgical technologists in the operating room. Their job is to help the surgeon and the scrub nurse to take care of you. A nurse or a surgical technologist wheels you from the waiting area to the operating room. Several people help you move from the gurney to the operating table. Because of light sedation, you may not remember all this activity. Later, when you are fully asleep, the nurses and the surgeon position you on the operating table.

The surgeon and the anesthesiologist accompany you to your surgical suite. The anesthesiologist makes sure that you do not feel pain and monitors your heart, lungs, and kidneys. This doctor inserts a needle into your arm so you can easily and quickly receive medications. Before putting you to sleep, the anesthesiologist attaches an oxygen monitor to your finger to measure your breathing during surgery. Once you are fully asleep, the anesthesiologist puts an endotracheal tube down your throat to prevent you from inhaling liquids into your lungs. It insures an open airway if you should need respiratory help during the operation.

While the anesthesiologist is working, the nurses wash and prepare your belly and pubic areas. To clean your skin they often use an amber-colored iodine-containing antiseptic and soap mixture. The surgical area must be thoroughly cleansed to prevent infections. Now you are clean and the nurses cover you with blue sterile drapes. To prevent you from becoming cold, they often enclose your upper body in a clear plastic jacket. Warm air circulates through the enclosed jacket to keep you warm. After stepping out to scrub their hands and arms, the surgeons enter the operating room. Surgeons are always assisted by colleagues, surgical assistants, or, when practicing in a university hospital, by resident surgeons. It often takes more than two hands to manipulate the complicated maze of sutures, clamps, and other surgical instruments. Surgical assistants, in addition to being an extra set of hands, are another set of eyes that help to make sure everything goes as planned.

Now it is time to get started. The surgeons are ready, the anesthesiologist adjusts the height and angle of the operating table, the surgical technologist hands the scalpel to your surgeon, and you, under a roomful of caring and watchful eyes, are on your way to regaining continence.

RECOVERY

At the conclusion of your incontinence and prolapse procedures the anesthesiologist stops the flow of anesthetic gas and removes your endotracheal tube. A few welcoming words bring you back to consciousness. You respond with a groan and slide back to sleep. Nurses move you from the surgical table to a transport gurney and then you are moved to the recovery area, where nurses monitor your blood pressure and other vital signs. A friend or family member may be allowed to sit nearby.

If you had a minimally invasive surgery such as bulking agent injections, then after recovering from the anesthesia, you may get dressed and go home to recover fully. You will need someone to drive you home, as you may be light-headed and possibly a bit fuzzy if you were given sedatives during the procedure. Do not make any major decisions for at least twenty-four hours after your surgery.

If you have had more extensive surgery, such as a retropubic procedure performed through an abdominal incision, then a nurse or nursing assistant will take to your hospital room. Once situated in your room, a nurse will give you hydrating fluids and pain medication intravenously. To prevent blood clots, your legs will remain covered in pressure cuffs until you are able to walk. It will be a few more hours before you are fully awake. Later, when you try to reconstruct events, you will discover that you do not remember much.

Major surgery can make the next few days slow and painful. Your doctor or a medical associate will come by to check your progress, to remove vaginal packing material, and to check your surgical wounds. Because you haven't eaten in a long while, food tastes terrible. However, in a few days your appetite will return.

Many women have difficulty urinating immediately after surgery and may have to go home with a bladder catheter in place or use self-catheterization. Usually the need for the catheter is gone within a week or two.

It is important to use pain medication even after you get home. Controlling pain will improve your recovery by helping you to move more easily and by preventing overwhelming exhaustion. Most patients require some prescription-strength pain medication for one to two weeks after their surgery.

To assure proper healing after incontinence and prolapse surgery, doctors recommend that "you take it easy." You should refrain from lifting more than eight pounds (the weight of a gallon of milk), driving, sexual intercourse, and exercise (other than walking) until your doctor says it is safe to do so.

Be sure to "listen to your body" and get enough rest, fluids, and, when your appetite returns, nourishing food. Taking advantage of pain medication also helps the recovery process by making walking less painful. This reduces your risk of forming blood clots and helps you to gradually regain strength and stamina.

Your ability to return to work depends on the type of surgery you had, your overall health, and the kind of work you do. Most doctors recommend that you stay home from work for one to six weeks to recover from major surgery and a week for the less invasive procedures. If your job involves extended physical activity, your doctor may recommend a longer leave of absence or limited work responsibilities.

Sexual activity after surgery is an emotionally laden subject. Some incontinent women have abandoned their sexual lives because they feared losing bladder control during intercourse. While it's common to feel a bit apprehensive after surgery, many women do return to an active and satisfying sex life.

Although occurring infrequently, there are some postoperative signs and symptoms that you should report to your doctor that may indicate infection or some other complication. These include:

- Prolonged feelings of urinary urgency
- Prolonged need for the bladder catheter
- Bleeding
- Foul-smelling discharge from the vagina or surgical wound
- Foul-smelling urine
- Increased abdominal pain
- Fever
- Back pain
- Nausea, vomiting, diarrhea, or constipation

A REALISTIC VIEW OF OUTCOMES

You hope your surgery will make bladder control "just like it used to be." Although research shows that these surgical procedures do help many women regain total or greatly improved bladder control, it takes time to recover from the surgery and to relearn brain-bladder control habits. It is also important to remember that incontinence surgeries do not help all women regain their desired degree of bladder control.

Immediately after surgery, some women report increased incontinence, urine retention, overactive bladder symptoms, and bladder muscle spasms. While for most women these problems are temporary, a few women will have permanent overactive bladder or urine retention problems. These are known risks of having incontinence surgical procedures. It is not possible to always predict who will have these outcomes even if the surgical procedure went well.

Before returning home from the hospital, some women may need to learn to self-catheterize to remove urine from their bladder. After getting home, others may need to resume their scheduled urination exercises to reeducate their bladder or use medication to calm bladder muscle contractions. Again, this is usually a temporary situation. On very rare occasions, women are unable to relearn how to urinate and for the rest of their lives have to use a catheter to empty their bladder.

Though satisfied with their results, many women report that urination after surgery is different. Their urine stream may be less strong and some women have to learn how to position themselves differently on the toilet (for example, leaning back) to urinate. This is because continence surgery purposely alters the relationship between the positions of the bladder and the urethra so that you do not leak. Unfortunately, this repositioning can sometimes make urination difficult or impossible. The very few women who have this problem after their surgery are either relieved because they are no longer wet, or are frustrated by catheter dependence.

It is natural to feel impatient to return to your normal activities after surgery. But you will need to give your body time to recover. It will take time to reestablish good brain-bladder communication. Your body needs to remember how to respond to normal urge signals and to learn appropriate responses to new messages.

After all your hard work with exercises, diet, medications, and more, it is natural that you want a cure. You no longer want to think about the bathroom all the time. But just like your original decision to have surgery, evaluation of surgical outcomes is somewhat subjective. Clinicians consider both total continence and improved continence as successful surgical outcomes. However, the factors involved in how they define success can vary depending upon the patient's satisfaction, the ability to restore total continence on a permanent basis, and restoring total continence for at least five years. These issues make it difficult to evaluate surgical research reports and to compare and contrast success rates for the different surgical procedures.

The fact that no two patients are exactly alike is another factor complicating efforts to compare surgical procedures and success rates. Many intertwined factors can lead to incontinence. Similarly, genetic predisposition, childbirth, athletic and workplace considerations, obesity, diet, and the long-term effects of other surgeries are all factors that contribute to surgery success rates for procedures to correct incontinence. Some factors result from the interplay between the surgical procedure and the patient's health. These may include the extent of pelvic floor damage, the combination and complexity of the surgical repair strategies applied on a case-by-case basis, as well as the patient's health and age. Other factors include healthcare quality issues such as the surgeon's experience and postoperative care. The patient's ability and willingness to follow recovery instructions is another important consideration. As you can see, evaluating the success of surgery is both complex and difficult.

As confusing as all of this may seem, there are many ways to improve your surgical results. Some treatment strategies involve medical care choices involving recommendations from your doctor or specialist. Others are entirely up to you. As we have said before, it is important to have a surgeon who is interested in and frequently performs female incontinence surgeries.

Then there are the things that only you can do to increase the likelihood of a successful surgical outcome. It is important to follow your doctor's postsurgical instructions regarding rest, lifting, work schedule, and other strenuous activities. It is also important to make lifestyle changes that are likely to promote good pelvic floor health and continence. These include maintaining a healthy body weight, eating a fiber-rich diet, drinking enough water, not smoking, performing pelvic floor exercises, and avoiding foods that cause bladder irritation (see chapter 4).

Like many other points we have discussed in this book, the decision to undergo incontinence surgery is a process. However, unlike patients who need to undergo emergency surgeries, you have the luxury to take the time to research and decide if a surgical approach to regaining continence is the right answer for you.

WORKSHEETS

Worksheet 9A: Choosing a Surgeon

The process of choosing a surgeon involves many objective, practical, and emotional decisions. While there are no "right" answers, this question inventory will help you to identify a surgical practice and a surgeon who will be a good working partner.

After answering these questions make a list of the items that matter most to you. Then review the list and decide which of these are the *most important* and which are nice, but not necessary.

Finding a Surgeon

The Surgeon

I would prefer to see a:
- ____ gynecologist who regularly performs incontinence surgeries
- ____ urogynecologist who specializes in incontinence surgeries
- ____ urologist who specializes in incontinence surgeries
- ____ general surgeon who regularly performs incontinence surgeries

I would prefer that my surgeon:
- ____ is in a solo private practice
- ____ is one of many surgeons in a group private practice
- ____ works in a university or regional medical center
- ____ no preference

I would prefer that my surgeon is:
- ____ male
- ____ female
- ____ no preference

My doctor's age is:
    ___ an important consideration
    ___ not an important consideration

English is not my native language and I would prefer that my surgeon:
    ___ speak to me in my native language
    ___ speak to me in English
    ___ not an important consideration

The Practice

The surgeon's office location is:
    ___ very important
    ___ moderately important
    ___ not important

That the office is accessible by public transportation is:
    ___ very important
    ___ moderately important
    ___ not important

The hospital where the doctor performs surgery is:
    ___ acceptable
    ___ not acceptable
    ___ no choice

Insurance

Is this doctor on your medical insurance plan?
    ___ yes
    ___ no
    ___ no, but I am willing to pay the difference

Does this doctor accept Medicare patients?

___ yes

___ no

___ no, but I am willing to pay the difference

First Impressions

The Office

After visiting the medical office, it appears that communication between the front office and medical staff is:

___ efficient

___ not efficient

___ not known at this time

After calling the medical office, it appears that working with the office phone system will be:

___ easy

___ frustrating

___ not known at this time

The office and medical staff is polite and respectful to patients.

___ yes

___ no

___ not known at this time

I feel comfortable in this office:

___ yes

___ no

___ not known at this time

The Surgeon

The surgeon:

    ___ listens and seems genuinely interested in helping me

    ___ does not listen to me

    ___ does all the talking

The surgeon:

    ___ is willing to provide his or her relevant training and surgical experience information to you

    ___ is uncomfortable about providing his or her relevant training and surgical experience information to you

    ___ would not provide information

The surgeon:

    ___ explains things clearly and fully

    ___ does not explain things clearly and fully, but has a good clinical reputation

    ___ makes me feel uncertain of his or her surgical skills

Worksheet 9B: Getting Ready for Surgery

Preparing for your downtime should not become an overwhelming task. The list below is a guide to make this task easier for you. Be sure to tailor it to your family needs. Encourage family members to participate in making the "to do" list. Remember to enlist the help of friends and family.

Use this list to organize your efforts and assure that you will have time to relax before going to the hospital.

Work

____ Inform appropriate individuals of your dates of absence
____ List those who need to know about your absence
____ Make arrangements with human resources office for sick leave

Home

Make a list of things that must be done
____ when it needs to be done
____ who should do it
____ designate a home "manager"

How to pay and when to pay
____ utilities, water, gas, electricity
____ charge cards
____ taxes

Banking and other money matters
____ legal cosigner, power of attorney
____ deposits
____ withdrawals
____ location of checkbook
____ permission to sign charge cards

Outdoor plant watering
___ where
___ when

Indoor plant watering
___ where
___ when

Lawn mowing and other yard work
___ when
___ where

Snow removal
___ name and phone number of snow-removal service
___ family members responsible for snow removal

Laundry
___ dry cleaners
___ location of cleaning supplies and washing machine instructions
___ folding and sorting

Dishes
___ dishwashing schedule

Pet care
___ when to feed animals
___ what do they eat

Mail
___ stamps
___ sending mail
___ bringing in and sorting mail

Garbage

    ___ pick-up day

    ___ usual time of pick-up

    ___ location

Recycling

    ___ what gets recycled

    ___ where to put recycled items at home

    ___ collection location

Light housekeeping

    ___ sweeping and vacuuming

    ___ picking up

Children's activities

    ___ day and time

    ___ locations

Grocery shopping—if necessary provide a sample grocery list

    ___ when

    ___ where

Food and kitchen

    ___ ask family members about food choices

    ___ stock freezer with homemade or purchased foods

    ___ make some sample menus

Make a list of important phone numbers that include:

    ___ close family members

    ___ close friends

    ___ neighbors

    ___ children's friends

    ___ taxi

    ___ your doctors

___ hospital numbers

___ pediatrician

___ veterinarian

___ take-out and delivery restaurants

___ cleaning service

___ work contacts

___ carpools

___ church and synagogue contacts

Worksheet 9C: Presurgery Questions

Although you will have probably already received answers to these questions from your surgeon or from other clinical staff members, going over this list will help reveal areas where you need to review or to request more information.

Questions for your doctor:

How long does the actual operation take?
When can I see my family?
How long will I be in the hospital?
When can I go back to work?
What can I do during the recovery period?
How long does it usually take to recover?
What are some of the common recovery problems?
What are the anticipated results of my surgery?
What is the likelihood I might need more surgery?

Questions for the office nurse:

When should I stop eating and drinking?
Do I need an enema? If so, how do I give myself one?
What about my required morning medications—for heart conditions, epilepsy, or diabetes?
What should I bring to the hospital?
What things should I leave at home?
What time do I have to be at the hospital?
Where is the surgery admission desk?
Where can family and friends wait?
Who should I call if I decide to cancel this elective procedure?

Worksheet 9D: Postoperative Questions

Questions for the hospital discharge nurse:

What signs and symptoms should I watch for?

How much can I lift?

When do I need to make a postoperative appointment with my doctor?

Can I take a bath or shower after surgery?

Can I go up and down stairs when I get home?

How do I get out of bed so it does not hurt so much?

What should I do if I have trouble using the catheter?

How long should I use pain medication?

How long should I use the catheter?

Who should I call if I am bleeding or have a fever?

When can I remove my bandages?

Questions for your doctor:

What is the best way to contact your office if I am having problems?

What kind of aches and pains are serious? What should I do if I experience them?

How can I better control temporary postoperative incontinence problems? How long might these problems last?

How often may I take pain medication?

What foods should I avoid?

How long do I have to take it easy?

When can I go back to work?

When can I resume my other usual activities?

When can I resume sexual relations?

FREQUENTLY ASKED QUESTIONS

1. Can I have another baby after having incontinence surgery?

The decision to have another baby is a personal one. However, most urogynecologists recommend that you postpone incontinence surgeries until you have had your last baby or have a cesarean delivery to protect your surgical repairs. The only exception to this general recommendation is pregnancy and mid-urethral sling surgery. According to the manufacturer, the polypropylene tape cannot withstand the pressures of a pregnancy. It is very likely that you will lose continence and require more surgery.

2. Why do I have to wait so long between my diagnosis and my surgery date?

There are many reasons why there is often a big time gap between your decision to have surgery and the event. The most important reason is that your doctor needs time to evaluate your health and to determine the best combination of surgical treatments. Other reasons are very practical. Operating facilities are busy places. Room scheduling must leave operating suites available for emergencies and specific types of surgeries. A room that can accommodate continence procedures may be available only once or twice a week.

3. After recovery from my surgery, do I still have to worry about lifting heavy objects?

It takes ninety days for scar tissue to mature and become strong. Most doctors recommend that you refrain from lifting heavy objects during your recovery period. Ask your doctor what would be a good postsurgical weight limit for you.

4. Why have my friends needed two or three bulking agent injection treatments to narrow their urethra and thereby improve their bladder control?

Research shows that women may require up to three injections to get maximal benefit from their bulking agent treatments. More than three injections is unlikely to result in additional improvement.

5. I am forty-five years old and considering a mid-urethral sling procedure to treat stress incontinence. Does anybody know if there are side effects associated with having a polypropylene mesh ribbon imbedded in my lower abdomen for potentially more than thirty or forty years?

Surgeons have used mid-urethral sling procedures for less than fifteen years. Although sling materials are tested for safety and potential toxicity, their long-term effects are not known.

6. If I already have a pacemaker, can I also receive sacral neuromodulation treatment?

Yes, having both a sacral neuromodulator and a heart pacemaker is safe.

7. What if my surgery doesn't work?

Unfortunately, sometimes that is the case. In fact, one out of three women who have one surgery for incontinence will have another in their lifetime. When that happens there are other alternatives that may help. If your surgery does not work, your surgeon can repeat the same procedure or try another type of procedure. If all else fails, surgeons can install an inflatable sphincter to give you better continence control. To urinate, the patient activates a small pump surgically placed in the labia, abdomen, or thigh.

8. My doctor is encouraging me to have prolapse surgery. I am beginning to believe that it might be a good idea to do it now while I am still young, rather than waiting to see if it gets worse. Do you think I should have the surgery now or wait?

Age is not the deciding factor. If your prolapse makes bladder control difficult or makes you feel uncomfortable, or if your doctor feels there is a medical reason to have surgery—then consider having the surgery now. If the prolapse is not bothersome, and does not protrude outside of the vaginal opening, then you are safe to do nothing or to try a pessary.

CHAPTER 10

TALKING AMONG FRIENDS

"Don't wait!"
Jeri—three weeks after surgery and
eight years of deciding what to do.

STORIES

At first it was a little difficult to find women to interview. Then, a lucky break! A volunteer reader for this book—one who just happened to be the neighbor who knows everybody—said reading these chapters made her feel so excited that she couldn't resist telling her friends what she had learned about urinary incontinence. Then, she said why she was interested in this topic— recalling her turning-point moment when she watched urine drip into her shoes while waiting in line at an airport bathroom.

Like many hundreds of thousands of women, this woman believed urinary incontinence—short of having surgery or taking pills—was just something you lived with. Many women are very excited to discover that simple things such as dietary changes, pelvic floor exercises, and even bladder diaries and scheduled urination exercises can make such a big difference in their lives.

It didn't take long for the word to get out. Soon we were contacted by women who said: "I heard you are writing a book about bladder control. Can I tell you my story?"

Talking to neighbors is different than interviewing urogynecology clinic patients. Unlike the clinic patients, many of these women did not know the differences between urgency and stress incontinence. Initiating conversation took a little practice and usually required asking, "Do you have the 'gotta go' problem or do you 'laugh and leak'?"

Women who had the "gotta go" problem often said that a prescription for "bladder pills" was the outcome of a single doctor appointment. Many who had "laugh and leak" difficulties wondered why their doctor wouldn't prescribe bladder pills for them. A few pessary wearers, though pleased with the results, were frustrated by the inconvenience of having to go to the doctor just to get their pessary cleaned. A few women talked about their successful surgeries. One woman discussed her decision not to undergo surgery—even though this means she has to wear disposable briefs.

The women you will meet shortly are based on real people. While each has a unique story to tell, you will discover that common themes run through their accounts. Perhaps you will even find yourself nodding in agreement over familiar and shared experiences.

CECELIA

"I have been dribbling for at least ten years. I haven't bothered to talk to my doctor about it because everybody my age dribbles. When I do manage to get a doctor appointment, I use the time to talk about real ailments like my arthritic neck. Besides, I know how to manage this. I never leave the house without first going to the bathroom. I stay home until my morning coffee runs through me and I don't drink anything—even if I am thirsty. When I go out, I am always on the lookout for a bathroom."

There Is Help

Many women who have bladder control problems believe urinary incontinence, like wrinkles, is a natural part of aging. That belief, along with embarrassment and the feeling that it isn't a "real problem," prevent women from seeking medical care.

Talking about bladder control helped Cecelia to see that urinary incontinence was controlling her more than she was controlling it. In addition to having to organize her day around bathroom needs, she also admitted to feeling thirsty most of the time.

Just hearing that urinary incontinence is a treatable condition motivated Cecelia to ask many questions. Our discussion quickly led to the benefits of pelvic floor exercises, dietary changes, pessaries, and even the possibility of talking to her doctor about her problem. Just before leaving, we reminded Cecelia about the importance of pelvic floor exercises. "Ladies," Cecelia said, "I am doing them now."

HELENE

"It started very suddenly when maybe two or three times a day I would have feelings of overwhelming and uncontrollable urgency. Just turning on the kitchen sink would do it to me. When it happened, I couldn't ever make it to the toilet in time."

Having unexplained urgency made it difficult for Helene to leave the house without worrying about having an accident in public. To prevent this from happening, she wore pads and made frequent trips to the bathroom to make sure that if she had an accident, it would be a small one.

One-Stop Treatment

Like many other women, Helene assumed losing bladder control was something every older woman had to endure. But unlike many, she did mention it to her gynecologist during her next annual exam.

Her doctor prescribed a drug-containing skin patch to control urgency. She also prescribed a vaginal estrogen cream saying it, too, would help. Helene says using these medications has almost entirely eliminated urgency episodes. Although she does have dry-mouth, she says that she takes other medications that also have this same side effect.

Helene has been using the skin patch for nearly three years. When asked if she would consider taking a break from it, she said, "I wouldn't dare."

Although medication helps many women regain bladder control, it is important to give dietary changes and behavioral methods (bladder diaries and scheduled urination exercises) a chance. Using these techniques, either by themselves or in combination with short-term drug treatment, helps many women overcome overactive bladder symptoms.

You may be curious about why Helene also uses estrogen cream. After all, research shows that hormone replacement therapy, though it helps with pessary comfort, doesn't prevent or treat stress incontinence and prolapse. So why did Helene's doctor prescribe estrogen cream to help alleviate overactive bladder?

As it turns out, doctors noticed that some bladder urgency patients, who also used estrogen creams to prevent vaginal thinning, did better than patients receiving traditional overactive bladder treatments alone. Although researchers have yet to confirm this curious observation, some clinicians do recommend using estrogen creams for this purpose.

LYNN

Even as a child, laughing and rough-and-tumble play with her brother caused Lynn to leak urine. "It wasn't much of anything, but it did happen." Lynn says she noticed her leaky tendencies became more of a problem shortly after menopause. "I just deal with it. I never leave home without wearing a panty liner and I know the location of every bathroom in town."

A recent annual checkup with her family doctor caused Lynn to think differently about bladder control. After her examination, the doctor told her that she had pelvic organ prolapse. He also wondered if she had bladder control problems. Lynn says that saying "yes" to that question was strange. "I had never put a name to it before."

Her family doctor suggested that she see a surgeon right away to repair the prolapse. "I didn't like that he wanted to push me into an operation so quickly, so I made an appointment with my gynecologist so I could learn more about this. Now, I wear a pessary and it works just fine."

Treatment Is a Process, Not a Quick Solution

Many women seeking stress incontinence treatment receive medication or surgery without having the opportunity to try simpler methods such as scheduled urination exercises or a pessary.

Not all women who have stress incontinence require surgery. Many find they can successfully manage stress incontinence by increasing the amount of dietary fiber and water they consume, regularly doing pelvic floor exercises, or by wearing a pessary. However, for some women, surgery is their only option for regaining bladder control. If this is your situation, remember surgical procedures are there to help those women who need them.

JUDITH

Judith, a new neighbor, is thirty years old. In addition to having a nine-month-old baby, she has two other young children.

"I leaked for nearly six weeks after the birth of my last child. My doctor said doing pelvic floor exercises would stop the leaking. Believe it or not, I actually told her that with three kids—plus my college classes—I just didn't have the time to do anything extra. Gee—what did I know! After she explained how to do them and that I could exercise virtually anywhere, I realized that what I said was pretty funny. Anyway—the exercises worked and the leaking stopped a few weeks later."

What Happened Here?

Not every woman who has bladder control problems is middle-aged or older. Many women experience temporary leaking during pregnancy and just after delivery. Usually, with recovery, the leaking stops within a few weeks. For those women whose post-partum leaking lasts as long three months, nine in ten of them still have symptoms five years later.

Doing pelvic floor exercises, *even if you do not leak*, is one of the most important things you can do. Performing these exercises on a regular basis helps strengthen pelvic floor muscles and may prevent you from having leaking problems later in life.

MARTY

As it turns out, Marty is a nurse and works in a women's incontinence clinic. In addition to working with clinic patients, she also runs the urodynamic-testing clinic.

"I was sixteen years old when I had my first baby. He was a big baby—over eight pounds—and here I was still a growing kid myself. After his birth, I noticed I leaked urine when I coughed or sneezed. The doctor said it would go away on its own. Well, it didn't."

In many ways, her story parallels the ones she hears every day. "At first, my urine loss wasn't too bad. I controlled it by crossing my legs as soon as I knew I was going to cough or sneeze." However, as you can well imagine, this coping strategy didn't always work. Sometimes she couldn't stop what she was doing to cross her legs and sometimes she couldn't cross her legs in time. Having stress incontinence made participating on a women's soccer team difficult. So, at the age of thirty-eight, she got an incontinence ring pessary so she could stay dry while playing.

About ten years later, Marty started to have uterine bleeding problems. "I decided to take advantage of the hysterectomy and to get a transvaginal tape at the same time. Wow—what a difference! I can cough, sneeze, and play soccer without leaking. The funny thing is—it took me nearly two years to get over the habit of crossing my legs!"

Pessary to Transvaginal Tape

Marty managed stress incontinence for most of her adult life. She wore a pessary for nearly eight years, and now has a transvaginal tape to support and position her urethra. While it is unusual to have had all of these experiences at such a young age, it is fairly common for women to transition from a pessary to surgery.

Just like Marty, many women make the switch when there is reason to piggyback a stress incontinence surgery with a hysterectomy or some other surgical procedure. Their reasons range from "why not" to the desire to get away from pessary care.

Other women decide to have surgery when ongoing pelvic floor changes make it difficult or impossible to wear a pessary. When this happens, surgery may be their best "next option" for regaining bladder control.

SUSAN

It took several years before Susan decided to undergo surgery for stress incontinence and pelvic organ prolapse. "At the time I was teaching high school and was managing okay. The bathroom was right across the hall from my classroom. I worried more about bowel control than I did about wetting myself."

"I went in for a sling procedure and some 'tightening up,' but once inside the doctor discovered that I needed more extensive repairs. The surgery, instead of taking two hours, took over five hours to complete."

Recovery was slow. "It took me at least six weeks before I was really up and about and at least another two or three months before I really felt like my old self. Intimacy was difficult and I had to use vaginal stretchers for a while. My daughter used to laugh about 'Mom and her box of sex toys.'"

Unfortunately, Susan experienced several postoperative complications. While this does not always happen, having them did make her recovery more difficult.

"It took me a long time before I could pee. I could feel it, but I couldn't do it." Susan believes that having to self-catheterize for a long time caused the stubborn infection that was ultimately responsible for her surgical wound reopening. "In some ways this was worse than the incontinence. By this time I was back to teaching and I had all these little drainage bags to deal with."

Now, nearly five years after her surgery, Susan says she is happy with the outcome and still continent. However, she reports that urination feels different than it used to. "I don't have much stomach muscle tone or feeling on my bottom. Sometimes I don't know when I am really done peeing."

Susan still sees her urogynecologist for regular checkups and by all accounts is doing very well. In spite of the difficult recovery, she wishes she hadn't waited so long to have this surgery. She is also very happy to report that she can cough, sneeze, and laugh without worry.

Surgery and Risk

No surgery is risk-free. The most common postoperative problems include reestablishing brain-bladder communication and postoperative infections.

Surgery is traumatic and it takes time to recover and to reestablish function. Sometimes, because of prolapse and nerve and muscle damage, not all women regain the level of function they had hoped to achieve. Susan says that even though things aren't perfect, surgery did improve her situation.

Infections are always a concern. Infections prolong recovery time, increase medical care costs, and may even cause death. Most of these infections happen when bacteria that normally live in or on your body manage to get inside your bladder or surgical wound. This can happen in the hospital or at home.

Self-catheterization is a common cause of postoperative infections. To prevent this from happening, many doctors prescribe antibiotics for their patients to take while having to "self-cath." Some women have difficulty relearning how to void on their own. This can lead to catheter dependence and ongoing voiding difficulties.

MARGARET

Margaret is seventy years old and is full of life. She participates in several quilting groups, belongs to a neighborhood book club, and because of arthritis and knee-replacement surgery goes to water aerobics classes six days a week. At the time of this interview, she had just returned from a weeklong camping trip.

Her leaking started about a year and a half ago. Laughing, coughing, sneezing, or getting up from a chair caused her to wet herself. As you know, these are classic stress incontinence symptoms.

She attributes her problem to having had five children in seven years. "Most of them were big babies and none of them just popped out." Then at the age of thirty-nine, she had a hysterectomy. "The doctor told me afterward that he did some other repairs and tightened me up."

After the leaking started she tried managing on her own. A few months later, a bout of kidney stones sent her to the doctor's office. "When I went to see the urologist, I told him about the leaking, too."

Kidney stone tests also revealed a problem with one of her ovaries. After recovering from that surgery she told her urologist, "No more cutting. The knee surgery was very hard on me, I take high blood pressure medication and I am also dealing with diabetes and now—kidney stones. Enough is enough."

The urologist sent her to a biofeedback specialist. The physical therapist, in addition to helping her with pelvic floor exercises, gave her disposable brief samples. After trying several styles, Margaret found the ones that worked best for her. Margaret says that wearing disposable briefs keeps her active without embarrassment. "However, I have to think more about going to the bathroom. I don't want to run off 'half-cocked.'"

Making Personal Decisions

As you can see, Margaret is juggling multiple medical problems. Some of them, such as diabetes and high blood pressure, require careful medical management. However, as we said in chapter 4, diet and medication scheduling adjustments may help her to improve bladder control.

Margaret's story is also one that illustrates the importance of good communication. By saying "No more cutting," Margaret is telling her doctor in straightforward terms what she wants for herself. By acknowledging this firm statement, the doctor helped her to "do the best she can with what she has" by referring her for biofeedback therapy.

While inconvenient and embarrassing, urinary incontinence is not a life-threatening condition. Margaret uses disposable briefs to manage her stress incontinence and is actively engaged with her family, friends, and community. Therefore, her choice to forgo an *elective surgical* procedure is a perfectly reasonable decision.

THE BIG PICTURE

Each year in the United States, nearly 3 million women give birth vaginally. Of these, anywhere between 30,000 and 180,000 will experience (usually temporary) bladder control problems during their pregnancy or afterward. By the time these 3 million women reach menopause, approximately 360,000 of them will have ongoing bladder control problems. While having vaginal delivery does increase risk for incontinence and prolapse, it is not the entire story. By age seventy-nine, nearly one in eight women—even if they had cesarean deliveries or are childless—will have had at least one incontinence or prolapse surgery.

The women you just met are a few of the many millions of women living their lives with incontinence. A generous bunch, they told you everything—from embarrassing moments to regaining sexual intimacy and successful recoveries. Because of them, you are not alone.

APPENDIX A

RESOURCE ORGANIZATIONS

Agency for HealthCare Research and Quality
P.O. Box 8547
Silver Spring, MD 20907
Phone: (800) 358-9295 and (410) 290-3841
Web site: http://www.ahrq.gov
A US government site that provides evidence-based medical practices information for clinicians and patients. Use this site to learn more about specific incontinence treatments and surgeries.

American Association of Retired Persons (AARP)
601 E Street NW
Washington, DC 20049
Phone: (800) 424-3410
Web site: http://www.aarp.org
A general resource for lifestyle, health, and healthcare information.

American Diabetes Association

1701 N. Beauregard Street

Alexandria, VA 22311

Phone: (800) 342-2382 and (703) 549-1500

Web site: http://www.diabetes.org

This nonprofit organization provides health and healthcare information for people who have diabetes. Use this site to learn how diabetes affects your overall health and how to best control your blood sugar.

American Foundation for Urologic Disease

1128 N. Charles Street

Baltimore, MD 21201

Phone: (800) 242-2383 and (410) 468-1800

Web site: http://www.afud.org

A site that contains links to an assortment of other urology Web sites. One such site—UrologyHealth.org—provides information for people who have various urinary tract disorders.

American Geriatrics Society

The Empire State Building

350 Fifth Avenue, Suite 801

New York, NY 10118

Phone: (212) 308-1414

Web site: http://www.americangeriatrics.org/

A professional association promoting high-quality, comprehensive, and accessible care for America's older population. The organization provides information on common diseases and disorders that affect older adults through its subsite: http://www.healthinaging.org/agingintheknow/

American Urogynecologic Society (AUGS)

2025 M Street NW, Suite 800

Washington, DC 20036

Web site: http://www.augs.org/i4a/pages/index.cfm?pageid=205
A professional organization that also provides information for
 patients with urinary or anal incontinence as well as pelvic
 organ prolapse. Use their site to find a local urogynecologist
 who performs incontinence surgery.

American Urological Association (formerly the American Foundation for Urologic Disease)

1000 Corporate Boulevard
Linthicum, MD 21090
Phone: (USA only) (866) RING AUA (866-746-4282) and (410)
 689-3700
Web site: http://www.auanet.org/index.cfm
Note: UrologyHealth.Org (http://www.urologyhealth.org/) is the
 American Urological Association's online patient information
 site.
A professional association for the advancement of urologic patient
 care. Web site features a patient information subsite.

Bladder Health Council of the American Foundation for Urologic Disease

1128 N. Charles Street
Baltimore, MD 21201
Phone: (800) 242-2383 and (410) 468-1800
Web site: http://www.afud.org
A site related to the American Foundation for Urologic Disease
 listed earlier.

The Continence Foundation

307 Hatton Square
16 Baldwins Gardens
London ECIN 7RJ
United Kingdom
Web site: http://www.continence-foundation.org.uk/

A product-sponsored site that provides information for people
who have bladder and bowel problems. Using this site will
help you learn more about bladder control management strategies and absorbency products.

The National Association for Continence (NAFC)
P.O. Box 1019
Charleston, SC 29402-1019
United States
Phone: (800) BLADDER (800-252-3337) and (843) 377-0900
Web site: http://www.nafc.org/
A nonprofit Web site features the Resource Guide of Products and
Services for Incontinence: a comprehensive index of all
known incontinence products and services available in the
United States and the Take Control Support Group Kit
designed to assist in development of a monthly support group
for women experiencing bladder control problems.

**The National Kidney and Urologic Diseases Information
Clearinghouse**
3 Information Way
Bethesda, MD 20892-3580
Phone: (800) 891-5390
http://kidney.niddk.nih.gov/
An information dissemination service of the National Institute of
Diabetes and Digestive and Kidney Diseases (NIDDK), which
is part of the National Institutes of Health (NIH). The Web site
features an A–Z list of topics and titles and easy to read publi-
cations. Also features information about clinical trials and
guidelines, including studies that are recruiting patients, clinical practice guidelines, and research reports.

National Women's Health and Information Center (NWHIC)
US Department of Health and Human Services

Office on Women's Health
200 Independence Avenue, SW
Room 730F
Washington, DC 20201
Phone: (800) 994-9662
Web site: http://www.4women.gov
A US government Web site that contains information and resource
   links to a wide range of women's health issues.

The Simon Foundation for Continence
P.O. Box 835
Wilmette, IL 60091
Phone: (800) 237-4666 and (847) 864-3913
Web site: http://www.simonfoundation.org
The mission of this nonprofit organization is to reduce the stigma
   of having incontinence and to provide help and hope to people
   with incontinence, their families, and the health professionals
   who provide their care.

Society for Women's Health Research
1025 Connecticut Ave., NW, Suite 701
Washington, DC 20036
Phone: (202) 223-8224
Web site: http://www.womenshealthresearch.org
The Society for Women's Health Research is a nonprofit organi-
   zation whose mission is to improve the health of all women
   through research, education, and advocacy.

Society of Gynecologic Surgeons
Web site: http://www.sgsonline.org/
A professional organization that also provides information for
   patients on the topic of surgical treatments for incontinence.
   You can use this Web site to find a surgeon who performs
   incontinence surgeries.

APPENDIX B

GENERAL READING

Newman, D., and M. Palmer, eds. "State of the Science on Urinary Incontinence." *American Journal of Nursing* (March): Supp. 2–57.

US Department of Health and Human Services. "The Public Health Implications of Urogenital Disease: A Focus on Overactive Bladder." *Clinician* 21, no. 4. http://www.4woman.gov/Health Pro/eduandasso/Clinician_5.pdf (accessed April 16, 2006).

READINGS BY CHAPTER

Chapter 1

"The Health Repercussions of Stigma." http://www.thepfizer journal.com/default.asp?a=journal&n=tpj37 (accessed August 16, 2005).

Chapter 2

Wagner, Todd, and T-W Hu. "Economic Costs of Urinary Incontinence in 1995." *Urology* 51, no. 3: 355–61.

World Health Organization. "World Health Organization Calls First International Consultation on Incontinence." July 1, 1998. http://www.who.int/inf-pr-1998/en/pr98-49 (accessed August 16, 2005).

Chapter 3

Freeman, R. M. "The Role of Pelvic Floor Muscle Training in Urinary Incontinence." *British Journal of Obstetrics and Gynaecology* 111, suppl. 1: 37–40.

Tubaro, A. "Defining Overactive Bladder: Epidemiology and Burden of Disease." *Urology* 64, no. 6: 2–6.

Chapter 4

Dietary Guidelines for Americans 2005. http://www.health.gov/dietary guidelines/dga2005/document/ (accessed August 23, 2005).

Chapter 5

"Knowledge, Attitudes and Practices of Physicians Regarding Urinary Incontinence in Persons Aged Greater Than or Equal to 65—Massachusetts and Oklahoma." *MMWR Morbidity and Mortality Weekly Report* 44, no. 40 (1995): 747, 753–54.

Chapter 6

Lynch, Darren. "Cranberry for Prevention of Urinary Tract Infections." http://www.aafp.org/afp/20041201/2175.html (accessed May 6, 2005).

Chapter 7

Rogers, R. G., D. N. Kammerer-Doak, and M. Spearman. "Obstetric Anal Sphincter Lacerations: An Evidence-based Approach. Part 1: Anatomy and Risk Factors." *Female Patient*. http://www .femalepatient.com/html/arc/sel/april02/article07.asp (accessed August 23, 2005).

Rudolph, W., and S. Galandiuk. "A Practical Guide to the Diagnosis and Management of Fecal Incontinence." *Mayo Clinic Proceedings* 77 (2002): 271–75.

Chapter 8

Burgio, K. "Influence of Behavior Modification on Overactive Bladder." *Urology* 60, no. 5, suppl. 1 (2002). http://www.ncbi .nlm.nih.gov/entrez/query.fcgi?cmd=Retrieve&db=PubMed& list_uids=12493360&dopt=Abstract (accessed August 23, 2005).

Diokno A., et al. "Prospective, Randomized, Double-Blind Study of the Efficacy and Tolerability of the Extended-Release Formulations of Oxybutynin and Tolterodine for Overactive Bladder: Results of the OPERA Study Group." *Mayo Clinic Proceedings* 78 (2003): 687–95.

Rogers, R. G. "Sexual Function in Women with Pelvic Floor Disorders." *Female Patient* 29 (2004): 30–38.

Chapter 9

Kammerer-Doak, D. N., and R. G. Rogers. "Surgery for Stress Urinary Incontinence Part 1." *Female Patient* 27, no. 10 (2002): 11–15.

Nilsson C. G., C. Falconer, and M. Rezapour. "Seven-year Follow-up of the Tension-free Vaginal Tape Procedure for Treatment of Urinary Incontinence." *Obstetrics and Gynecology* 104, no. 6 (2004): 1259–61.

Nygaard, I. E., and M. Heit. "Stress Urinary Incontinence." *Obstetrics and Gynecology* 104, no. 3 (2004): 607–20.

Rogers, R. G., and D. N. Kammerer-Doak. "Surgery for Stress Urinary Incontinence Part 2." *Female Patient* 27, no. 11 (2002): 10–16.

GLOSSARY

Anal incontinence: Involuntary loss of bowel contents including gas, liquid, or solid stool.

Anatomy: Organs, tissues, and structures that make up the body.

Anticholinergics: A class of medications used to reduce muscle spasms and cramps.

Antihistamine: A type of medication used to treat rashes, itchy eyes, and runny nose symptoms we associate with allergies and colds. Some people make more urine as a side effect of taking these medications.

Anus: The outermost opening of the lower intestine. Normally, the anus remains tightly closed until the appropriate time to have a bowel movement.

Apex: The peak or uppermost region such as the highest part, or top, of the uterus.

Atrophy: The breakdown and loss of muscle tissue that can be caused by lack of muscle use, disease, or severe physical damage. Atrophy or thinning of nonmuscle tissue can also result from disease or severe physical damage.

Bacteria: Microscopic organisms that sometimes cause infections.

Biopsy: A small piece of tissue that a doctor removes and checks for signs of disease.

Bladder capacity: The amount of fluid your bladder can comfortably hold.

Bladder compliance: The ability of the bladder to stretch while maintaining low pressures.

Bladder stress test: A test that evaluates if coughing causes you to leak urine.

Caffeine: A naturally occurring substance that may cause feelings of agitation and is also a bladder irritant.

Catheter: A thin tube used to transport liquid in or out of body organs.

Constipation: The condition when having a bowel movement is difficult or infrequent (less than two times each week). Taking certain medications, consuming a low-fiber diet, and not drinking enough water can cause constipation.

Contraction: Tightening and shortening action of a muscle.

Contrast media: A liquid that contains substances that x-rays do not pass through. Using contrast media produces light and dark areas on the x-ray film and increases the ability to see anatomic details.

Cysto: Any word beginning with the prefix "cysto" has something to do with the bladder.

Cystocele (or anterior compartment defect): A weakened point in the support of the upper vaginal wall support. This weak point can allow the upper vagina wall, with the bladder and urethra following, to sag toward the vaginal opening or even slide partially out through the opening.

Cystometrogram: A bladder test that allows you to report urge sensations as your bladder fills with water—literally means measuring (metro) and recording (gram) the pressure in your bladder (cysto) as it fills with fluid.

Cystoscope: An instrument that consists of a miniature camera, a thin fiber-optic tube, and an intense light source that allows the doctor to examine the inside of your urethra and bladder.

Cystoscopy: Using a cystoscope to look inside your bladder.

Detrusor: Three layers of muscle that together form the bladder wall.

Diabetes: The condition when people can no longer efficiently use the glucose molecules contained in simple sugars and carbohydrates. Having large amounts of glucose in the blood causes people to produce large amounts of urine, which can worsen incontinence.

Diaphragm: An arched platform of muscle that lies between the abdominal cavity (which includes the intestines, bladder, and reproductive organs) and the thoracic cavity (which includes the lungs and heart).

Diuretic: A food substance such as caffeine or a medication that causes people to make more urine. Sometimes people call these medications "water pills."

Elective surgery: A voluntary procedure that improves health but is not a lifesaving surgical procedure.

Endotracheal tube: The tube the anesthesiologist places down your throat to help you breathe.

Enema: A fluid used to clean out the bowels.

Enterocele (or apical compartment defect): A weakened area on the top (apex) of the vagina that may cause the vagina to turn inside out like a sock and protrude outside the body. With severe prolapse, the small bowel, the bladder, the rectum, and the uterus are contained within the vaginal protrusion.

Episiotomy: A surgical cut made between the lower opening of the vagina and the anus.

Estrogen: A female hormone.

External anal sphincter: Anal sphincter muscles that contract when we cough or sneeze. This muscle is under our control. It relaxes when we have a bowel movement and contracts when we perform pelvic floor exercises.

Fast or **fasting**: To go without eating for a prescribed time.

Fiber: The indigestible parts of fruits, vegetables, and grains.

Fistula: A hole or tunnel that develops between adjoining body cavities.

Gastrointestinal: Referring to the stomach, intestines, and other organs involved in digestion and excretion.

Glucose: A type of sugar.

Gurney: A bed with wheels.

Healthcare Provider: A general term used to describe all types of healthcare professionals.

High blood pressure: When the pressure in your arteries is too high both when your heart pushes blood out or rests between beats.

Immune system: A coordinated group of body organs and cells that help protect us from invading bacteria, viruses, and other microbes.

Internal anal sphincter: The anal sphincter muscle controls moment-to-moment anal continence. This muscle is not under voluntary control and is normally "closed" or contracted.

Laparoscope: An instrument that enables the doctor to look into the abdominal and pelvic cavities through a small incision.

Ligament: A sheet of tough and fibrous tissue that connects or supports bones, muscles, and pelvic organs.

Menopause: The natural process of gradual hormonal changes that result in a permanent end to women's reproductive cycles. Menopause usually begins when women are between the ages of forty-five and fifty.

Mid-urethral sling: A surgical procedure in which a meshlike ribbon of tissue or manmade material is woven under the mid-portion of the urethra to reposition and support the urethra, to prevent bladder leakage.

Narrow angle glaucoma: Short-term eye pain resulting from an increase in eye pressure.

Nervous system: The network of nerves that rapidly transmits signals to and from the brain.

Neurological: Functions associated with the network of nerves that carry messages, in the form of electrical impulses, throughout the body.

Neuromodulation: Using drugs, electricity, or electricity-generating implants to make therapeutic changes in nervous system activity.

Nocturia: Urination urge sensations occurring during the night to the degree that they cause a person to awaken.

Nocturnal enuresis: Urination while asleep.

Nurse Midwife: A practitioner who specializes in women's healthcare including the delivery of babies.

Nurse Practitioner: A nurse who has completed specialized training beyond nursing school.

Off-label medications: Medications people use in ways that are different than those described on the label.

Overactive bladder: A condition in which miscommunications within the normal nerve pathways between the brain and bladder cause the detrusor muscle, or bladder wall, to contract abnormally (too frequently and/or too forcefully), thus signaling the need to urinate even though the bladder is only slightly filled.

Overactive bladder, dry: Overactive bladder symptoms of frequent and/or forceful urgency sensations occur without the unplanned loss of urine.

Overactive bladder, wet: Overactive bladder symptoms of frequent and/or forceful urgency sensations occur accompanied by the unplanned loss of urine.

Oxalate: A naturally occurring substance, found in many foods and beverages, that can sometimes cause bladder irritation.

Pelvic cavity: The space encircled by the pelvic and pubic bones and the lower back bones.

Pelvic floor: A hammock-like network of muscles that form a supportive "floor" in the base of the pelvic cavity. The pelvic floor muscles support the correct position of organs and help control bladder and bowel functions.

Pelvic floor exercises: Also called "Kegel" exercises, after Dr.

Arnold Kegel, the physician who discovered the importance of exercising this muscle group. These exercises involve contracting the muscles that support the urethra, bladder, uterus, and rectum.

Pelvic Inflammatory Disease (PID): An infection of the pelvic organs including the fallopian tubes, ovaries, and uterus that may ultimately cause infertility.

Pelvic organ prolapse: When the vagina and the pelvic organs behind it slide down and protrude outside the body.

Perineum: The tissue between the vagina and the rectum. Childbirth often causes perineal tears.

Pessary: Small, flexible, and removable silicone rings that are placed inside the vagina to help support the pelvic organs and prevent leaks.

Physical Therapist: Someone who specializes in treating the muscles and connective tissue problems in the body.

Physician's Assistant: A healthcare professional who has completed an in-depth medical curriculum and is licensed to practice medicine as a healthcare team member with physician supervision.

Polypropylene: A type of plastic.

Postvoid residual: The amount of urine remaining in your bladder after you urinate.

Postvoid residual test: A measure of how well you can empty your bladder.

Puborectalis: The sling-shaped muscle that stretches behind the rectum, which when contracted, can kink the anal canal to prevent stool from passing through it.

Rectocele (or posterior compartment defect): A weak point in the support of the bottom vaginal wall. This weak point can allow the vagina walls, with the rectum behind it, to sag toward the vaginal opening or even slide partially out through the opening.

Rectum: The end of the lower intestine, where stool is stored before it is pushed out of the anus during a bowel movement.

Reflex arc: Involuntary physical reaction caused when nerves stimulate tissues in more than one area.

Retropubic: Behind the pubic bone.

Saline: Salty water.

Sedative: A medication that "quiets" or "calms" specific target organs such as the heart or brain.

Self-catheterize: When the patient uses a catheter to empty their bladder.

Speculum: A metal or plastic instrument used to hold open the vagina during a gynecological examination.

Staging: This is when clinicians evaluate medical conditions and compare them against research-validated standards. Each stage associates a standardized "score" to the changes present.

Stress incontinence: Unplanned loss of urine, usually occurring with laugh, cough, sneeze, or physical exertion, which creates increased abdominal pressure on the bladder, causing urine to be forced out through the urethra.

Stretch receptors: Nerve endings that send signals to the brain as a result of detecting muscle tissue stretching.

Sutures: The material the surgeon uses to sew tissues together or the process of sewing tissues together.

Tranquilizer: Medications that make people feel calm without putting them to sleep.

Transobturator tape (TOT): A mid-urethral sling procedure in which a meshlike ribbon of tissue or manmade material is woven under the midportion of the urethra to reposition and support the urethra, serving to prevent bladder leakage. Surgical incisions are made just below your pubic bone and the ribbon is threaded through the naturally occurring holes located on both sides of your *pelvis*.

Transvaginal tape (TVT): A mid-urethral sling procedure in which a meshlike ribbon of tissue or manmade material is woven under the midportion of the urethra to reposition and support the urethra, serving to prevent bladder leakage. For this procedure, two very small incisions are made in your lower abdomen just above your pubic bone and a third incision in the vagina provides access to the urethra.

Ureters: Two tubes that carry urine from the kidneys to the bladder for storage.

Urethra: The tube that extends from the bladder neck to carry urine out of the body.

Urethral sphincter: The muscular region at the junction of the urethra and bladder. It remains tightly closed to keep urine in the bladder and opens when you urinate.

Urogynecologist: A doctor who specializes in treating women for urinary and pelvic floor disorders.

Urologist: A doctor who specializes in treating problems with men and women's urinary systems.

Vagina: The tubelike cavity between the lower end of the uterus (womb) and the opening at the vulva (outer lips) of the female genitals.

Vaginitis: A general term to describe vaginal swelling, burning, and itching usually resulting from having a vaginal infection.

Valsalva maneuver: A brief action of breath holding and bearing down often used to help have a bowel movement or speed up urination. It is capitalized in honor of Antonio Valsalva (1666–1723), the Italian doctor who identified the action.

Vesical pressure: The total pressure exerted on bladder contents.

Void: To empty the bladder when urinating.

White blood cells: Infection fighting cells.

INDEX

f = figure   *t* = table   *w* = worksheet